KU-827-396

Contents

Introduction

The low-FODMAP diet is a highly researched front-line treatment for irritable bowel syndrome (IBS) that is based on solid science. Developed by Monash University in Melbourne, Australia, back in 2006, the initial excitement came when a landmark study showed amazing symptom relief for about 75 per cent of people with IBS.[1] Since its conception, a wealth of research has shown this diet can help bring relief from symptoms including bloating, diarrhoea, abdominal pain and flatulence. This is huge news for the IBS world, as these symptoms really can affect quality of life. We had been aware for some time that certain foods, like onions, broccoli, cauliflower and beans, could be IBS triggers – now we had the science to explain how and why! Nutrition news travels fast, and the evidence backing it up is so good that the low-FODMAP diet is included in the clinical guidance for IBS treatment in countries around the world, including the USA, Canada, New Zealand and the UK. Leading research is now being carried out at Monash University as well as King's College London, UK, two institutions that have championed the low-FODMAP diet. There is now plenty of evidence showing the low-FODMAP diet can reduce IBS symptoms in 50–80 per cent of patients with IBS.

> **What are FODMAPs?**
>
> **F**ermentable
>
> **O**ligosaccharides
>
> **D**isaccharides
>
> **M**onosaccharides
>
> **a**nd
>
> **P**olyols
>
> These are short-chain carbohydrates that are poorly digested by the body.

The low-FODMAP diet has three stages, and the aim is to reduce or even relieve symptoms while enjoying foods that are as varied as possible. One of the big misconceptions with this diet is that it's all about restriction, but that is only the first stage, so let's bust that myth straight away. The aim is ultimately to enable you to expand your diet, as we know that eating a varied diet is good for your overall health, your gut health and your social life, too, enabling you to eat out without stress and enjoy different kinds of food!

Another misconception is that the low-FODMAP diet is something you should use as an initial treatment for IBS. There are actually other strategies to try first – then, if these have not had adequate effect, you move on to the low-FODMAP diet. Sadly, many people are given a diagnosis of IBS and sent home with instructions to google this diet and follow whatever advice they find on the internet – and this advice can often be very conflicting, sometimes even going against clinical guidance. In this book I take you through the initial diagnosis and the first-line advice that you should explore first. Then, once you have a clearer idea of whether it could help you, we will move on to the low-FODMAP diet.

On the surface, the diet sounds simple: cut out foods that are known to be problematic, wait a few weeks for your symptoms to settle down, then reintroduce the foods and see which ones give you problems. In practice, it is more complicated. Maybe you are one of those people who have been told to go away and research the low-FODMAP diet on your own. If so, you will know that there is a wealth of information out there, and that it's often contradictory and confusing. Why? Well, we are all individuals, and this is very much a diet that should be tailored to your needs. That's the role of a dietitian. It was never designed to be a diet you could follow using the advice of Dr Google. This is a restrictive diet that brings with it risks of nutritional deficiencies, an impact on the gut microbiome (the bacteria and microorganisms that live in your gut) and a lot of work. However, it is also a diet that can have huge benefits for some people, reducing symptoms and improving quality of life. This books sets out to clear away some of the confusion, but it is my aim that you use this knowledge while working alongside a FODMAP-trained dietitian. In fact, the main IBS guidelines recommend a dietitian is always involved. Most doctors are not trained specifically in nutrition, and certainly not in nutrition for IBS. Not all dietitians are trained in this, either. You wouldn't ask a plumber to lay a patio: choosing the right specialist to support you is important if you want to get a good outcome.

The low-FODMAP diet does not cure IBS, but it does provide good symptom relief for about 75 per cent of patients (although this does also show that some will sadly get no benefit).[2] This is worth bearing in mind as you go through the process. The low-FODMAP diet is often touted as a magic cure, but in reality it does not work for everyone. Sometimes, the initial advice, which is so often skipped over, is what can really help. That's why we'll be starting at the beginning and covering it all. Even if your symptoms do not completely disappear, hopefully they will become more tolerable – and by learning about your triggers, you will find ways to manage your condition.

1. WHAT IS IBS?

I BS, or irritable bowel syndrome, is just what its name suggests. It's a condition where your gut becomes irritated, and symptoms including bloating, abdominal pain, excess wind, diarrhoea and/or constipation ensue. Sadly there is no magic cure, but there are tricks and techniques to help you manage the condition.

IBS falls under the umbrella of functional gastrointestinal disorders (FGID). These are the most common gut conditions, affecting one in five people, and can be challenging to manage as there are few medications that will just solve the problem. Functional gastrointestinal disorders can be trickier to diagnose as there are no real tests: diagnosis relies on examining the symptoms reported and excluding other conditions, so it can be quite subjective. Other functional bowel disorders include functional diarrhoea, functional constipation, functional abdominal bloating and unspecified functional bowel disorder. These conditions are described as 'functional' because they cause changes in the function of the gut, without any physical features such as ulcers, inflammation or thickening of tissue.

The symptoms of IBS can feel very debilitating and can affect your quality of life, as well as leading to multiple trips to your doctor. Symptoms and concerns about the condition can lead to people avoiding socializing, finding themselves unable to eat out, planning their lives around toilet trips or struggling with their attendance at school or work. Getting things under control is therefore important. No one wants to be constantly worrying about where the nearest toilet is, whether they will still fit into their clothes at the end of the day, or if they are going to spend an entire evening out with friends struggling with abdominal pain. Fortunately, there are dietary and lifestyle strategies that can help. While this brings hope, the process can be a lengthy one, so medication and coping strategies are very much part of the plan, too.

IBS symptoms involve abdominal pain with altered bowel habits: this can be diarrhoea, constipation or both. IBS with diarrhoea (IBS-D) is the more common variant. Up to nine out of ten sufferers report that food gives them symptoms, so you can see that diet has a huge impact.[3] While IBS does not increase the risk of mortality, it certainly has an impact on quality of life and has a huge cost to healthcare systems.

IBS is often diagnosed between the ages of twenty and thirty, with 5–12 per cent of the worldwide population suffering.[4,5] More women seeming to be affected than men (14 per cent of females and 9 per cent of males).[6] Despite being a fairly common condition, it can often go undiagnosed with people just seeing their symptoms as something they need to live with. IBS can also be one of those labels you are given when nothing else quite fits your symptoms. Rather than being a made-up condition or something to 'put up with', this is a lifelong disorder that can really affect your quality of life. A large survey reported over 78 per cent of people with IBS said their condition affected their day to-day-lives, including travel, eating out and physical relationships.[7] The longevity of IBS means there are also lots of older people suffering who may not have been diagnosed before, or who have been living with IBS for some time. If you know someone like this, do encourage them to seek treatment, as there is new research coming out all the time, offering fresh hope.

Your symptoms and treatment can change over time, so even if you have tried using dietary treatments in the past to no avail, I'd heartily recommend you try again. The first step is to see your GP and get that diagnosis.

Diagnosis of IBS

Common symptoms of IBS

Common symptoms of IBS include lower abdominal pain and discomfort, bloating and changes in bowel habits. Some people can also suffer from heartburn, nausea and feeling full quickly. Other symptoms include excessive wind, tiredness, incomplete emptying when passing a bowel motion, an embarrassingly noisy stomach that gurgles (known as borborygmi) and pain in the rectum. These symptoms are not there all the time, but they tend to follow a pattern through the day or week. There can be times when they are worse, and other times when things are more settled. Often a period of high stress will be the trigger to symptoms flaring up.

You should be assessed for IBS if you have had any of the following symptoms for six months or longer:

- abdominal pain or discomfort
- bloating
- change in bowel habits [8]

Symptoms of IBS: a summary

Symptom	Description
Bloating	Increased pressure in the abdomen.
Distension	Change in the circumference of the abdomen.
Abdominal pain	Visceral hypersensitivity (extra-sensitive nerve endings in the gut) or cramping of the gut wall.
Diarrhoea	Too much fluid, inflamed colon, too-fast movement through the colon.
Constipation	Too little fluid, slow transit along the colon, too much dry matter.
Altered transit time	If foods are moving faster or slower through your bowel that usual.
Increased wind and flatulence	It is perfectly normal to pass wind 7–14 times a day, or 20 times a day for some people. If you feel full of gas a lot of the time, or flatulence is causing social issues for you, then it may be abnormal.

It is important that you do not jump in and attempt to diagnose yourself. While it may appear that your symptoms are obvious, it is vital that you ask your doctor to thoroughly examine you to rule out other, more serious conditions that have similar features to IBS. Coeliac disease, diverticular disease, endometriosis, pancreatic disorders, pelvic floor disorders, inflammatory bowel disease, some autoimmune disorders and certain cancers can all have overlapping symptoms, so these must be checked for. Take a look at the list of 'red flags' below: these are warning signs that suggest you may have a disease or condition other than IBS. If you have any alarm bells or feel you have not been properly assessed, then do chat to your GP.

Red flags

Signs that your symptoms may be something other than IBS include:

- symptoms starting after the age of fifty
- blood in the stools or rectal bleeding
- fever
- unexplained weight loss (of more than 5kg/11lb)
- waking at night for a bowel movement
- family history of colorectal cancer or bowel diseases
- IBS in a first-degree relative (such as a parent, a child or a sibling)
- coeliac disease in a first-degree relative

- existence of another autoimmune condition (e.g. type 1 diabetes, lupus, rheumatoid arthritis)
- persistent daily diarrhoea
- recurrent vomiting

If you have any of these symptoms, please let your GP know.

How IBS is diagnosed

IBS is officially diagnosed and defined through using the ROME IV criteria.[9] This can seem a little complicated, which is another reason why it is important not to self-diagnose. First, you should have had abdominal pain for at least one day a week for the past twelve weeks. Over the past three months, you should have abdominal pain that passes after a bowel movement, or abdominal pain that is associated with a change in bowel habits (going more or less often, or a change in the form of your stool). All symptoms should have started at least six months ago for a diagnosis of IBS to be made. The diagnostic criteria is summarized in the table on page 12.

A simpler way to think about this is the ABC criteria:

- **A**bdominal pain
- **B**loating
- **C**hanges in bowel habits

You may also experience additional symptoms, including:

- an altered stool passage (straining to pass a stool, feeling an urgent need to open your bowels for a poo, or a feeling of not having fully emptied your bowels – this is known as 'incomplete evacuation')
- abdominal distension (an increase in the size of your tummy)
- symptoms that are aggravated by eating
- mucus in your stool
- back pain, tiredness, nausea and bladder issues

Certain medications can also cause symptoms that are similar to IBS. For example, antibiotics can cause an upset tummy, codeine and iron supplements can be the cause of constipation, and metformin can lead to diarrhoea, nausea and abdominal pain. Some typical tests that are usually carried out before a diagnosis is made include: a full blood check, a blood test to look at your C-reactive protein levels, checks on the nutritional markers in your blood, faecal calprotectin levels and a blood test for coeliac disease (this test needs to be done at time when you have been regularly eating gluten for six weeks). While it can be tempting to pay privately for additional tests, do be cautious, as many do not have the science behind them to back them up, which means the results can be confusing. For example, microbiome tests, IgA food intolerance tests, intestinal permeability tests and anything like saliva, hair or energy-level tests can be wildly inaccurate and will not give you easy-to-interpret answers. If these tests worked consistently and it was this easy, the NHS would be using them.

Diagnostic criteria for IBS: a summary

You must have had this for at least one day per week over the past three months	Recurrent abdominal pain relieved by having a poo or associated with a change in bowel movements
Plus at least two of these symptoms regularly over the last three months: **1.** Change in stool habits (straining, urgency, incomplete emptying) **2.** Bloating **3.** Symptoms worsen after eating **4.** Mucus in your poo	• abdominal pain related to a bowel motion (having a poo) • change in the frequency of passing stools • change in the appearance of the stool

Adapted from NICE (The National Institute for Health and Care Excellence) guidelines.[10]

Understanding bowel movements

A question I am often asked is: 'What is a normal bowel movement, and how often should I be having one?' So, let's get on to the subject of poo!

Stool features are a very important part of IBS diagnosis. Think about the shape and texture. Ideally you want a 'smooth sausage', a number four on the stool chart below. Pellets or stringy stools can mean constipation, while loose stools suggest diarrhoea. It can be usual to pass some mucus at times, but blood in your stool is always a reason to see your GP. How often you empty your bowels is something that varies from person to person, so get to know how your own bowels work. Not everyone will do a poo on a daily basis.

It can be normal to poo between one and three times a day, or even just three times a week. The key is knowing what is normal for *you*. Then you can assess if and when you see changes in your bowel habits.

Stool chart

Use this chart to assess what your bowel habits are like.

Type 1		Separate hard lumps, like nuts (hard to pass)
Type 2		Sausage shaped but lumpy
Type 3		Like a sausage but with cracks on the surface
Type 4		Like a sausage or snake, smooth and soft
Type 5		Soft blobs with clear cut edges (passed easily)
Type 6		Fluffy pieces with ragged edges, a mushy stool
Type 7		Watery, no solid pieces, entirely liquid

Q: How often should I do a poo?

Do not be concerned about talking to your doctor or dietitian about your poo! We are used to it, and it really will not phase us. Stool frequency varies from person to person, so try to work out what is usual for you. Going less than three times a week or more than three times a day is usually considered abnormal.

Types of IBS

While the term IBS is often the diagnosis people are given, the reality is that it is more complicated than this. There are several types of IBS, and the type you have will influence what advice works for you. So always bear that in mind. If you do not feel that you fit into one category, it is worth chatting to your GP about whether you do actually have IBS, to make sure you receive the right treatment. For example, if you do not have abdominal pain, but do suffer from lumpy stools, incomplete evacuation and have fewer than three bowel movements a week, it is more likely you have functional constipation.

Types of IBS

IBS with predominant constipation (IBS-C)	You have stool types 1 or 2 more than 25% of the time, and stool types 6 or 7 less than 25% of the time.
IBS with predominant diarrhoea (IBS-D)	You have stool types 6 or 7 more than 25% of the time, and stool types 1 or 2 less than 25% of the time.
IBS with mixed bowel habit (IBS-M)	You have stool types 1 or 2 more than 25% of the time, and stool types 6 or 7 more than 25% of the time.
IBS unclassified (IBS-U)	You meet IBS criteria, but your bowel habits do not meet any of the three groups above.

What causes IBS?

The simple answer is we just do not know: there is no single cause. However, there can be some risk factors and triggers that can lead to IBS symptoms worsening.

1. An oversensitive gut. Many of the symptoms seen in IBS are due to visceral hypersensitivity. This means some people have a digestive system that is extra sensitive to the processes of digestion and also that bacterial fermentation can trigger their symptoms. The nerves in the digestive system can also be more sensitive, making gas or water retention feel more painful, and leading to increased bloating. There can be changes in the speed at which food moves through the gut, leading to it moving faster (diarrhoea) or slower (constipation). Some people may have low-grade inflammation or experience changes in the immune system, making it more reactive.

2. Genetics. Studies on twins show that if one twin has IBS, it is more likely the other twin will have it too, and we know that IBS can occur in more than one family member. This does not mean there is necessarily a genetic link, however, as environment also plays a role. If you live in the same house and eat the same foods, you will also share the same gut bacteria. However, neither the genetic nor the environmental factors mean that just because someone in your family suffers from IBS, you automatically will too.

3. Gut infections. A study following a waterborne pathogen leading to severe diarrhoea led to many people exhibiting a higher risk of IBS. Specifically the results showed a four-and-a-half-fold increase in the risk of IBS two years after the infection, and a three-fold increase in risk after eight years.[11] This is known as post-infectious IBS. In a similar way, some people can develop IBS after a bad episode of gastroenteritis, food poisoning or after courses of powerful antibiotics.

4. Anxiety and stress. There is a well-known link between stress in the brain and the gut, with IBS being more common in people suffering from anxiety or depression. While it can feel frustrating to be told to work on your stress management when you know there is a digestive issue, this really can help. Many people will notice their gut symptoms are worse during stressful periods. Your enteric nervous system is a collection of neurons in the intestine that you can think of as the brain of your gut. This interacts with your actual brain. When the brain is stressed, it can stress the gut via this gut–brain axis. For some people, a traumatic event or period of severe stress can be the trigger for IBS.

5. Gut microbiome. An imbalance of bacteria in the large intestine may contribute to IBS symptoms. When some foods are poorly digested and absorbed they will pass into the colon, where the bacteria break down the food fragments further in a process known as fermentation. Gases are released as by-products. This process is totally normal and happens in all of us, but some people are more sensitive to it and their gut symptoms can be triggered.

6. Dietary triggers. This is what we will come on to talk about later in this book (see pages 36–7).

IBS symptoms in more depth

Let's have a little anatomy lesson. The digestive system, in its simplest form, is a series of tubes. The food moves from the mouth, down the oesophagus, into the stomach, then into the small intestine, where it is broken down and some is absorbed. The leftovers move into the large intestine (the colon), where more nutrients are absorbed, and then the remainder is packaged into stools. The arrival of faeces into the rectum signals the urge to pass a poo. The rectum should contract and the anal sphincter should relax. In IBS, this overall system doesn't work as effectively as it should – or it works too effectively! Let's take a look at the main symptoms in more detail.

The digestive system

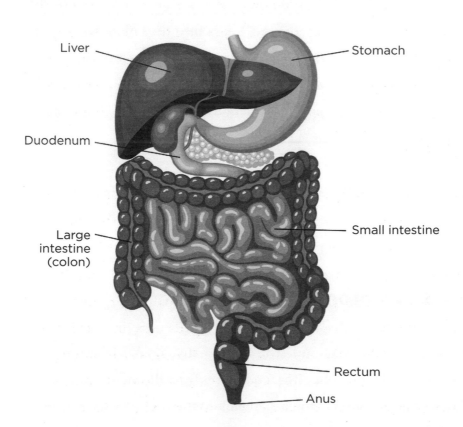

Liver

Stomach

Duodenum

Small intestine

Large intestine (colon)

Rectum

Anus

Bloating and distension are often just lumped together under the term 'bloating'. In fact, bloating is a change in the *pressure* felt in the tummy, while distension is a change in the *size* of the tummy. Distension of the small and large intestines is a common symptom caused by solids, liquids and gases, and this can lead to pain, the uncomfortable sensation of bloating and the visible distension seen.[12] Some people describe being a couple of clothing sizes larger after meals or feeling 'pregnant'. Typically, bloating and distension will be at their worst after your largest meal of the day, which for many people is in the evenings. It is important to remember that bloating is a normal part of digestion and is meant to happen: it is the degree to which it happens, and the pain it causes, that is the issue in IBS. For some people, the bloating may not look severe, but they might have more sensitive nerve endings in the intestine, making it feel very painful.

Changes in bowel habits can be varied, depending on the type of IBS you suffer from. Diarrhoea is when there is more water in the bowel than matter. Either there is too much liquid coming in, the colon is inflamed and not able to dry out its contents or things are just moving through the intestines too quickly. There are some foods that we all absorb poorly. These foods pass into the large intestine, but they take water with them to help them pass through. This excess fluid is then expelled, leading to that loose stool. Some people have more gut sensitivity than others, and may have a gut that moves things through at a faster rate. Constipation, on the other hand, can be due to too little fluid, too much drying out of the matter in the bowel or the muscles not moving things along quickly enough, resulting in bloating and distension. Some people will alternate between constipation and diarrhoea on different days. Getting to know your normal bowel habits is useful, so keep a diary of how often you do a poo and what consistency it is. Take a look at the stool chart on page 13, and remember that type four is the 'perfect' poo, smooth and sausage-shaped. See also pages 39–45 for advice on fibre, as fibre and fluid can be key to helping your bowels.

Transit time links in with the changes in bowel habits described above. It is the speed at which matter moves through the bowel, from one end to the other. This is affected by your enteric nervous system. Some people will naturally have a longer transit time and open their bowels a few times a week, while for some people it will be faster, and they will poo two or three times a day. A faster transit time is seen in 15–45 per cent of people with IBS-D, while in those with IBS-C, 5–45 per cent have a slower transit time. Altering the time it takes for food to pass through your system can improve your IBS symptoms. The key is to know what is normal for you. Too little fibre can slow things down, while a large amount of poorly absorbed sugars may lead to quicker, more explosive movement. It is worth noting that certain medications can slow down transit time (for example, narcotics and codeine), as well as well as iron supplement tablets. Do chat to your doctor if you are concerned about this.

Abdominal pain is a common feature of IBS. How much pain is felt depends on the sensitivity of the nerve endings in the gut. If these are very sensitive, it is known as visceral hypersensitivity. Doctors can test your visceral hypersensitivity by inserting a tube with an inflatable balloon attached to it into the rectum. People with IBS have been shown to experience greater discomfort when the balloon is inflated, and can tolerate less inflation. Probably not something to try out at home! More sensitivity to this distension causes more pain. Abdominal pain can also be a result of contractions of the muscles in the gut wall, causing cramps.

Gas production occurs as the bacteria in the large intestine feed on unabsorbed food molecules. This is called fermentation, and the by-products are a range of gases, including butyrate and propionate, and short-chain fatty acids. Some people experience greater levels of gas production than others, and some people are more sensitive to the gas. They may have gut bacteria that are faster fermenters and greater gas producers. Some people are better able to move the gas down and out of the body through flatulence, whereas for others that gas can sit around, creating discomfort.

Wind and flatulence are totally normal! We can pass wind 7–14 times a day, expelling up to 2 litres of gas a day. If you feel are you passing gas too frequently, then reducing your FODMAP intake may help. The smells from flatulence are something we would all like to avoid, and these can be worse in IBS. These smells can originate from bacteria fermenting protein, which happens when there is more protein than carbohydrate around. Maybe you are eating more protein than you need, or you are eating fewer carbohydrates, so there is more protein there as a result. While you may not like having to pass wind, it is important to 'let it go', as otherwise the gas will be held in your large intestine and can lead to further abdominal pain and bloating.

How do foods cause your symptoms?

With 60 per cent of IBS patients reporting symptoms get worse after meals, specifically within 20 minutes of eating, and 93 per cent reporting symptoms being worse within three hours of eating,[13] it is clear food plays a key role in IBS. Studies show 70–89 per cent of patients with IBS report that foods trigger their symptoms, and they therefore limit or exclude foods as a result. The long-term plan is to be able to eat as diverse a diet as possible, so you do not want to be cutting out foods for good unless you definitely know they are a problem for your body. The best way to test for foods causing gut symptoms and food intolerances is to exclude them from your diet and then reintroduce them. It's not as high-tech as a test, but it's the system that we know works, and it's the process we'll be exploring in this book.

Q: Do I have a food allergy?

While some people may talk about food allergies in IBS, this is not common or accurate. The terms food allergy and food intolerance are often used interchangeably, but they are not the same thing. Food allergies are less common and are reactions to proteins in the food, leading to an immune response. The body makes antibodies and histamine is released when the food allergen and antibodies meet. Some of these allergic reactions can be tested for using skin-prick tests. Food intolerances or hypersensitivities are more common, and do not involve the immune system. They don't lead to the production of antibodies, making it harder to test for them. While there are tests marketed as being able to assess food intolerances, in reality they do not give an accurate answer, and can just add to the confusion about which food is causing the issue.

Understanding FODMAPs

Carbohydrates are chains of sugar molecules that are broken down by the digestive system into glucose in order to give us the energy we need. Some carbohydrates are poorly digested or absorbed. This is a normal process in all of us, but as we've learned, some people have a more sensitive gut than others. We call these difficult-to-digest carbohydrates FODMAPs (fermentable oligosaccharides, disaccharides, monosaccharides and polyols).

They pass along the digestive system, drawing water with them as they move into the large intestine, where they meet with billions of bacteria. The extra water that has been drawn along can lead to watery stools (hello, diarrhoea!).

The large intestine is where fermentation happens. The bacteria there feed on the FODMAPs and food particles. While small in size, the bacteria cause large side effects: gas and bloating. Often people with IBS produce more gas than others.

FODMAPs are found in a range of foods, including fruits, vegetables and wholegrains. In chapter 3 we will explore FODMAPs in more detail, including which foods contain them in high, moderate and low amounts.

Other factors

Additionally, some people may react to food chemicals such as caffeine, salicylates, glutamate (MSG), colourings and preservatives.

Your eating pattern can also have a huge impact. Eating too large a meal in one go, skipping meals and the amount of fibre you eat can all affect your symptoms. Failing to chew your food well, or not taking the time to sit down and eat your meal in a calm environment, can affect how your body digests the food. And let's not forget that those stress levels can play a role, so if you are feeling stressed, your digestive system may react in a different way.

Q: Why don't we all have IBS
if we all eat FODMAPs?

- *Everyone eats FODMAPs and produces gas as a result, but some people are more sensitive than others.*
- *Some bodies make more gas that others. This depends on the types of bacteria in your gut, as some bacteria produce more gas than others.*
- *The amount of bloating you experience depends on the sensitivity of your gut nervous system (enteric nervous system).*
- *Some people move gas out of their bodies faster than others.*
- *When the bowel bloats, the stomach muscles should tighten to stop the tummy distending too much. For some people, this happens to a greater degree than for others.*
- *Stress and anxiety can make us more sensitive to our gut signals.*

Initial treatment for IBS

Once you have seen your doctor and have a clear diagnosis of IBS, you can start working through the IBS treatment stages. While there are some drugs that can help alleviate symptoms, these are limited and there is no one magical medication that will cure IBS. The drugs that are available often come with side effects, which is one reason why many people will choose to use diet and lifestyle measures to help manage their symptoms. IBS is a lifelong condition, and taking medications long-term is not always how people want to deal with it.

As we've seen, it is not just diet that affects IBS symptoms: this really is a whole body and mind approach. Stress and anxiety can be key triggers. Techniques including yoga, meditation, cognitive behavioural therapy (CBT), exercise and gut-related hypnotherapy may also help you. Therefore, it is key to have a systematic approach to your treatment. I know you just want to get better, and it is tempting to jump in and try everything at once, or just dive straight in to the strategy you think will benefit you must, but you really do need to start at the starting line. That starting line is the 'first-line' advice outlined in the next chapter. It can seem too simple and even a bit patronizing, but so often in clinical practice we find it helps. For some people, making these simple changes can be the answer to helping their symptoms. If you can find a solution by making smaller, less drastic changes that work quickly, that has to be a good thing. So before you jump into cutting out food groups, please take some time to try the first-line advice and tips. IBS is like a jigsaw puzzle: you want to put together the edges first, then work through the middle, one piece at a time. Only once you have worked through the first-line advice will it be time to move on to the low-FODMAP diet.

The stages of IBS treatment

IBS diagnosis from your GP

Following a clinical assessment as well as a dietary and lifestyle assessment, including looking at your personal and family medical history, and carrying out blood tests and tests for coeliac disease (see pages 7–13).

Work out your IBS subtype

IBS-C, IBS-D or IBS-M (see page 15).

Keep a food and symptom diary

Follow the first-line advice (see Chapter 2)

Work through all the advice listed and monitor your symptoms. If this has not had enough of an effect, then consider if the low-FODMAP diet is right for you and if you have the time to commit to it right now.

Find a dietitian to support you

See pages 86–9 for more information about why this is a key part of the plan.

Stage 1 (4–8 weeks): Restriction (see Chapter 4)

Restriction or elimination of FODMAPs for 4–8 weeks. Swap high-FODMAP foods for low- and moderate-FODMAP foods, while monitoring your symptoms to see if this helps reduce them.

Stage 2 (6–12 weeks): Reintroduction (see Chapter 5)

Reintroduce FODMAPs and test your responses. This takes up to ten weeks. If you did not get any relief from your symptoms in stage 1, then the low-FODMAP diet has not worked for you, and it is time to go back to your healthcare team to look at other options, such as SIBO (small intestine bowel overgrowth) testing or revisiting the initial tests you had done. If there was symptom relief, then it is time to start reintroducing high-FODMAP foods to find out which ones are your personal triggers. Each FODMAP group is tested individually and symptoms recorded.

Stage 3: Personalization (see Chapter 6)

Now you know which FODMAP groups you can tolerate, and how much, it is time to include all well-tolerated foods in your diet, only restricting those that cause you symptoms. This stage can take a little tweaking as you work out your personal tolerance to foods containing more than one type of FODMAP (see page 158) and to combinations of different FODMAPs within a meal or a day. It is important to check you are meeting all your nutritional needs now, and to keep on reviewing this as things change over time.

Retest foods you enjoy at regular points in case your tolerance changes

2. FIRST-LINE ADVICE

Many IBS sufferers will already be aware that certain foods cause them more symptoms (alcohol, caffeine and spicy food are common culprits), while other foods are easier on their digestive system. However, there is no simple test to show what you should exclude, as it can be different for everyone. Instead, you need to test things out yourself. Have a look at the following tips and think about your current lifestyle.

Think about how you eat your meals

While this sounds very simple, eating is something many people rush through. Taking time over your meals, sitting at a table, away from distractions including work and screens, focusing on what you are eating and letting your brain and gut connect are all really important. Think about memorable meals you've enjoyed – perhaps on holiday, or at a restaurant. What makes them different? How does the experience compare to the way you eat at home? We have busy lives, which can mean eating on the run, grabbing lunch at your desk, or just not taking long enough to properly chew and digest. When you plan your day, make sure you also plan in time to sit down and eat. Block out that lunch break in your diary.

Remember to chew

Take the time to chew your food well. The average number of chews needed is estimated to be around 30 per mouthful. This may seem like a lot, especially if you are a quick eater, so try making a conscious effort to take longer over your meals. Of course, this will depend on the type of food. Soft, liquid foods like yogurt and soup will not need as much chewing, while harder or tougher foods, such as nuts and meat, may need more. Now, I'm not advocating that you start counting each chew, but it is a reminder to slow down and chew each mouthful well.

Don't skip meals

Skipping meals can leave you feeling extra hungry for the next meal, and this can encourage you to eat more, and faster, which is harder work for your digestive system. Planning your meals and making time for them in your schedule is key. It may be tempting to skip meals if you feel that certain foods are causing your gut symptoms, but doing so can actually worsen symptoms, while also making it hard to meet your nutritional requirements for nutrients like fibre.

Smaller meals can be helpful

This may mean you need to eat more frequently throughout the day in order to satisfy your hunger and meet your body's needs. A common source of bloating can be not eating much in the day, but then making up for it with a large serving of food in the evening. With a big load of food to digest in one go, it is not surprising if you feel bloated. It may also be that your serving sizes of certain foods groups are too large: this can be the case with carbohydrate foods, such as rice and pasta. Keep a food diary for a few days to help you assess how spread out your meals are and what your portion sizes are like. Do you need to adjust your meal timings, add in a snack or adjust your portions? You can check food labels to get an idea of the normal portion size for most foods. Eating a smaller portion may help your symptoms, but please do ensure that you still eat enough to nourish your body across the day: paying attention to your hunger levels is the best way to assess this. Remember to put your phone and any work away and take time to enjoy your meal.

Meal timings

Eating regularly throughout the day means you will need to structure your meals carefully. You may need to get up ten minutes earlier to make time for breakfast, or schedule a lunch break into your diary. Eating late at night can also be a trigger for IBS symptoms. In the hours before bedtime, your digestive system slows down, meaning you may be more likely to suffer symptoms at this time. Try having your evening meal earlier and planning in a lighter evening snack before bed.

Stress at meals

Try to keep stress away from the dining room. It may be helpful to use some breathing exercises before and after a mealtime to calm your nervous system. Think about what would make your mealtime environment more pleasant: maybe you could have something nice to look at on your table, a list of happy conversation starters or some calming music in the background. If you feel anxious or on edge after a meal, take 10 minutes to do a meditation exercise or read a book.

Five-finger breathing

This is a great way to help you reduce anxiety before meals – or at any time. To begin with, do this for 5 minutes, then increase as you get more used to it. Hold out one hand, then use a finger from your other hand to trace around the thumb and each finger of the hand you are holding out. Breathe in as you do this, then trace back from your little finger to your thumb as you breath out. Practise breathing deeply and see if you can add a short hold of the breath at the end of your inhale.

Introducing mindfulness

Mindfulness is focusing on being aware of the present moment, while calmly acknowledging and accepting your feelings, thoughts and bodily sensations. You can practise this while out for a walk. Often we walk with a purpose to get to a destination, usually in a hurry. Instead, try to connect with your body and surroundings. Take time to notice what you can see, hear and smell. Notice your thoughts and how your body feels. Take time to think about how the earth feels under your feet as you walk, how your arms swing, how your head, neck and shoulders feel. You could also stop to pick up some natural objects, like leaves, stones and sticks. Take a moment to examine them, really noticing the small details and connecting with nature.

Mindful meditation

After a meal, find somewhere quiet and comfortable to sit. Focus on your breathing, taking deep breaths in and out (you could use the five-finger breathing technique opposite if that helps you). Notice any thoughts you have, and let them pass. It is normal for thoughts and feelings to pop up. Try not to pass any judgement on these thoughts and feelings – just bring yourself back to focusing on your breathing. You may want to close your eyes or focus on an object. Some people also find holding an object helps them, while others like to play meditation music in the background. Try a few methods and find the one you like the most. As before, begin by practising mindfulness meditation for 5 minutes, and slowly build time up.

Discover your trigger foods

Spicy foods

Spicy foods, such as chilli sauce, cayenne pepper, curry and Tabasco sauce, can lead to an increase in IBS symptoms, especially in those who suffer with IBS-D (see page 15). Capsaicin, which is found in hot peppers and chilli, can speed up the movement of food through the digestive system, and can cause abdominal pain and burning sensations.[14] It is also worth thinking of the other foods in a spicy meal that may contribute to your symptoms, such as garlic and onions. People with a hypersensitive digestive system have been found to have more of a certain type of receptor that responds to garlic and spicy foods (known as TRPV receptors). This makes them more sensitive to these foods.

Fat

Some people with IBS have a lower tolerance for fat. You may notice you have bloating and pain after high-fat meals, or that the meal seems to sit in your system for longer. This is because fat prolongs the amount of time it takes for food to be moved through the large and small intestines. Reducing your fat intake, or spreading it out over your day rather than having a larger load in one meal, may help your IBS symptoms.[15]

Polyols, including sorbitol and xylitol

These are artificial sweeteners found in some sugar-free foods, including chewing gum and certain drinks. They can have a laxative effect, so if you chew a lot of gum, that could be one of your triggers.

Think about your fluid intake

Water

Fluid can help improve the passage of stools through the system and reduce the need for laxatives. Water is always the best option, but you could also try herbal teas (avoid chamomile, oolong, chai, fennel and dandelion teas). No-added-sugar squash (without polyols) can also help, or try adding some fruit to your water for flavour. Aim to drink 1.5–3 litres (2¾–5¼ pints) a day.[16]

Alcohol

Alcohol can induce or worsen the symptoms of IBS. It affects the motility of the gastrointestinal system, including how fast food moves through it. For some people, binge-drinking (having more than four drinks in one go) leads to loose stools, abdominal pain, nausea and indigestion. That alcoholic tipple can reduce absorption of nutrients from food and increases the intestinal permeability.[17] While the evidence we have is limited, it suggests up to a third of people find alcohol affects their IBS symptoms. So, limit your intake to moderate levels of no more than 1–2 units a day, with several alcohol-free days in your week. You could try some of the alcohol-free spirits that are now available. Limiting your consumption of alcohol to mealtimes will also help reduce the effect it has on your gut symptoms.

Caffeine

Caffeine can worsen IBS symptoms in some people. It is a stimulant and can make the digestive tract work faster: it increases the amount of gastric acid secreted and the speed at which food is moved through the colon.[18] There are not many studies in this area, but the evidence we do have suggests that some caffeinated drinks may increase constipation, while others may lead to loose stools. So have a think about the impact on your body on days you drink more caffeinated drinks compared to caffeine-free days. It is recommended you stick to a maximum of no more than three medium mugs of normal-strength coffee or four cups of tea a day (400mg caffeine). If you are pregnant, then halve this. Remember, caffeine is also found in hot chocolate, some energy drinks and chocolate bars, too.

Do you eat enough fibre?

Dietary fibre is one of the cornerstones of IBS management, but it's a controversial and confusing topic. Even the main guidelines we have for IBS disagree, because the research has such varied results. Some studies in IBS have shown that fibre neither helps nor hinders gut symptoms, while other studies show some moderate evidence in favour of fibre supplementation. It's all quite confusing, and finding the right approach for you can take some careful experimentation or an expert dietitian's eye. This makes the question of how to alter your fibre intake quite a tricky one, and it can take time to find the right balance for your body. It is something I would definitely encourage you to work on, though, as fibre has so many benefits. Diets rich in fibre are associated with a lower risk of cardiovascular diseases, stroke, type 2 diabetes and colorectal cancers.[19] Fibre can also help our gut bacteria, giving them food to munch on and ferment. Generally, it is recommended that we aim to eat 30g fibre a day, but this needs to be balanced with the fact that high amounts of fibre can also trigger IBS symptoms. If your fibre intake is lower than 30g per day, increasing it may help with constipation. Add fruit, vegetables, oats, beans, pulses and wholegrain cereals to your diet, but make sure you increase your fluid intake at the same time.[20]

See the 'How to eat more fibre on the low-FODMAP diet' table on pages 122–4 and the information alongside it for more information. Going from eating very little fibre to suddenly eating lots of it is not a good plan. Large increases in your fibre intake can cause symptoms such as bloating and abdominal pain. As with most dietary changes, you want to make small, sustainable adjustments that you can stick to in the long term.

Where is fibre found?

Fibre is found in wholegrain foods, including brown rice, buckwheat, oats, quinoa, potato skins, wholegrain breakfast cereals, wholegrain pasta and wholemeal bread. It is also found in nuts, seeds, beans, pulses, fruit and vegetables. This can make plant-based diets higher in fibre, and sometimes it is this higher amount of fibre that is causing some symptoms. Whether you eat a plant-based, vegan or vegetarian diet, or eat meat and fish, tracking your fibre intake over a few days can be a very useful indicator.

Soluble and insoluble fibre

There are three main qualities that impact how fibre works: solubility, viscosity and fermentability. Solubility is how well the fibre dissolves in water; viscosity is its ability to thicken in water; and fermentability is related to how it feeds the gut bacteria. The terms soluble and insoluble fibre are actually now being phased out, as most foods contain a mixture of both. However, in clinical practice, in books and on the internet, you will find most people still use these terms, as they are easy to understand and we need a simple way to classify fibre.

Certain fibres (including oats, apples, strawberries, lentils, psyllium, peas and barley) have a higher solubility. This means they dissolve better in water. These fibres increase gastric emptying, so things move faster, and they can help to lower blood cholesterol as well as helping to sustain blood glucose levels. Other fibres act like more of a bulking agent: they do not dissolve and are indigestible. These insoluble fibres act like a broom, helping to sweep out the digestive system, and passing into the large intestine for fermentation. Quinoa, kale and raspberries are examples. We need a balance of all types of fibre, which generally means you should focus on eating your wholegrains, fruits, vegetables, nuts and seeds. For example, eating more oats, peanuts, sesame and sunflower seeds can help you make a more fully formed, sausage-shaped poo. If you need help with more regular motions, try increasing your fruit, vegetable and wholegrain consumption. Take a look at the 'Types of fibre' table on pages 44–5 for your fibre needs. Remember you may need to experiment a little to see what helps.

Q: *What about resistant starch?*

Do you ever feel bloated after heating up last night's pasta for lunch? That could be due to resistant starch. This is a form of starch that resists digestion in the small intestine. Instead, it passes into the colon and can then trigger symptoms. It's found in reheated grains, rice, pasta, and potato, unripe bananas, and seeds and pulses. A common culprit can be takeaway rice.[21]

Constipation top tips

- Eat five portions of fruit and vegetables a day.
- Try flaxseeds. Begin by taking 6g (1 tablespoon) a day with a 200ml (7fl oz) glass of fluid. Increase this gradually over a three-month period up to 24g (4 tablespoons).
- Try eating more oats for a softer stool.
- Slowly increase your fibre intake from wholegrain foods if you do not have a high-fibre diet. Try oats, wholegrain rice, nuts and seeds.
- If you eat plenty of wholegrain high-fibre foods, try reducing these for a couple of weeks.
- Psyllium husk, methylcellulose or partially hydrolyzed guar gum are soluble fibre supplements that can be used for extra fibre.
- Keep drinking fluid – aim for about 2 litres (3½ pints) a day.
- Avoid extra wheat bran.
- Eating two kiwifruit will provide you with lots of fibre (one third of your daily intake), and can help with constipation – but you need to eat the skin as well. Give them a wash first.
- Rest your feet on a small stool when you are on the toilet and lean forward so you are in a semi-squat position with your hands resting on your thighs and your knees higher than your hips. This helps the pelvic floor to relax, and helps the anal sphincter to open.

Diarrhoea top tips

- Reduce your fruit intake to three portions a day, eating just one portion at a meal or snack time.
- Make sure you replace lost fluids: keep drinking around eight glasses of water a day.
- Reduce your caffeine intake to a maximum of three cups of coffee (or three to four cups of tea) a day and cut out any fizzy drinks.
- Try reducing your intake of insoluble fibre, for example from wholegrain foods and high-fibre supplements. Remember this is a short-term change.
- Try taking psyllium husk.[22]
- Avoid sugar-free foods, including sugar-free sweets, mints and chewing gum. The mannitol, sorbitol and xylitol these often contain can be a trigger.
- Use meditation and mindfulness as a way to reduce your body's overall stress levels (see pages 34–6).

Types of fibre

Fibre category	Foods	Actions
Type 1: Medium solubility, medium viscosity, low–medium fermentability	• psyllium • oats	• faster transit time • water holding • can help form a better-shaped stool that holds together
Type 2: Insoluble, non-viscous, non-fermentable	• all green plant cell walls • celery stalks* • stalks of leafy green veg • rhubarb • fruit and vegetable skins • peanuts* • almonds* • walnuts* • chia seeds* • pumpkin seeds* • sesame seeds*	• help with stool bulking • gel-like properties to help form stool • best for IBS-C (see page 15) • faster transit time
Type 3: Soluble, viscous, fermentable	• fruits • vegetables • legumes • guar gum • fenugreek • oats • Benefiber® Healthy Balance	• increase the production of short-chain fatty acids in the colon • help to form a better stool

Fibre category	Foods	Actions
Type 4: Soluble, non-viscous, fermentable	• flaxseeds • inulin • beans and pulses* • onions* • garlic* • artichokes* • wheat* • rye*	• can increase the growth of beneficial bacteria • increase the production of short-chain fatty acids in the colon

*These are all high in FODMAPs, so are not allowed during the restriction stage of the low-FODMAP diet.

Should I try pre/probiotics?

Probiotics are live bacteria that, when ingested in large enough amounts, can alter the overall balance of the gut bacteria (microbiome) in a positive way. Prebiotics are the foods for these gut bacteria and microorganisms. Some FODMAPs are prebiotics, including onions, garlic and wheat. If you do not have enough beneficial probiotic bacteria in your gut, this could part of the reason why you are suffering. These probiotic, healthy bacteria feed off the food that passes into the colon and ferment it, releasing gases. While this sounds like a negative process, it is actually very natural and happens to us all. However, for some people suffering from IBS, there is an imbalance in the levels of beneficial bacteria that could affect your symptoms. So it makes sense to look after your gut bacteria.

It would be wonderful if all you needed to do was take a test to assess what bacteria is present in your gut, and could then be told which supplement to take to top you up to healthy levels. Sadly, we are not yet there with this science. Microbiome tests do exist but they are not yet accurate enough for daily clinical use. They are also very expensive, plus your gut bacteria can vary over time, so the situation in your microbiome could change. There is research showing us that taking probiotics may help with IBS, but this is limited. However, it does make sense that feeding your gut with beneficial bacteria and food for those bacteria could be helpful.

So, which one should you take? The issue here is that there are so many strains of probiotics that we just don't always know. It is difficult to know which individual strain of probiotic bacteria your gut needs, so you may have to try a couple out. That being said, there is some limited evidence suggesting the following types of probiotics may be more useful to try if you have IBS.

- Activia yogurt taken once a day may help with constipation.[23] This study was carried out on women over a four-week period. It could be that other types of yogurt would also help, so consider including a live, natural, Greek or probiotic yogurt in your daily meal plan.
- Symprove is a liquid probiotic that has been shown to reduce symptoms over a 12-week trial.[24]
- Alflorex is a probiotic that has some evidence of reducing symptoms after four weeks.[25]
- VSL 3 is another probiotic that may help with flatulence.[26]

Before rushing out to buy one of these probiotics, I would recommend you talk it through with your dietitian first. New research is always coming out, and there could be something better suited to your specific symptoms. When trying probiotics, you need to give them some time to have an impact. This should be a minimum of two weeks, but you should ideally take them for four weeks and see if there is any improvement. If you don't see any benefits, you can try another strain – or it could be that the probiotic route is not one you need to go down. Check you are trying all the other first-line advice too.

While prebiotics are also something that the gut bacteria need in order to be fed and well, most of them are also high in FODMAPs, so this is something to think about later in your IBS journey if you embark on the low-FODMAP diet. Eating prebiotics can help feed the gut bacteria, and these specific foods can also selectively increase the beneficial bacteria (*bifidobacteria*). While you may need to reduce certain prebiotics if you eat follow the low-FODMAP diet, it is important to add some of these back into the diet later, in a staggered approach, to help you build up your tolerance (see pages 139–53).

Other approaches that could help

Medications
Medications can have some limited impact in helping the symptoms of IBS and are worth trying, so please do chat to your GP about

these. There are drugs to help with diarrhoea, as well as medications and natural remedies for abdominal cramps and bloating, such as peppermint oil and Mebeverine. Sometimes, an antidepressant may be helpful for reducing your stress. This is not something we will cover in depth in this book, but do chat to your GP about it.

Psychological approaches

Psychological treatments, such as CBT and hypnotherapy, can be helpful for some people with IBS. Your GP can refer you for psychological treatment if you have not responded to medication after 12 months.[27] Stress and anxiety can be big triggers for IBS, and psychological therapies can help to reduce these symptoms. The app Nerva provides a six-week psychology-based programme that you can use yourself at home.

Yoga

Yoga is another option that can help some people.[28] An analysis of six trials showed yoga decreased bowel symptoms and improved quality of life. We need more research to confirm this, but mindful activities, including yoga, Pilates and tai chi, are known to help reduce stress, calm the mind and help you feel connected to your body. They are definitely worth a try.

Q: Should I go gluten-free?

There is some evidence that a gluten-free diet can give symptom relief in some people with IBS-D who have specific genotypes, but this is a small group. Other studies show no benefits at all. Why is this? Well, cutting out gluten may appear to help, as you are also reducing wheat, which is a FODMAP. Gluten is just better known as being potentially problematic.

Q: If I exclude foods, will I be deficient in nutrients?

A study showed that IBS patients who excluded foods still had similar daily nutritional intakes to the general population. This may be due to an increased awareness around nutrition and health, so try to focus on eating a balanced diet. If you are cutting out foods, it is important to ensure you replace the nutrients in those foods. If you have any concerns, chat to a dietitian for advice.[29]

First-line advice: summary

Only once the approaches outlined in this chapter have been tried should the next stage be attempted. These first-line treatments are so much easier to incorporate into a busy lifestyle. However, if they have not worked, then it may be time to find a specialist dietitian to help you with the low-FODMAP diet.

The following table summarizes the first-line advice. Refer back to it and monitor your reponses to these changes as you make them.

This is worth reviewing at different points in your monthly cycle for women, and also at times when you are feeling more or less stressed and anxious.

First-line advice

Make time for meals	Set time aside in your day to eat, sit away from your work and enjoy your meal. Eat slowly and chew well.
Reduce stress before meals	Stress can affect your digestion, so take some time to breathe deeply and reduce your anxiety before starting on the food.
Eat small, frequent meals	Eating smaller meals (if you normally have larger meals) can help. This may mean you need to eat more snacks between meals to respond to your hunger and meet your body's nutritional needs.
Reduce your alcohol intake	Drink no more than two units of alcohol per day, with some alcohol-free days.
Reduce your caffeine intake	Stick to three mugs of coffee or four cups of tea a day (400mg caffeine). If pregnant, reduce this to 200mg.
Reduce spicy foods in your diet	Try reducing spicy foods to see it this helps.
Reduce the fat content in your diet	If you tend to eat a lot of fat, reducing your consumption of it may help.

Alter your fibre intake	• Avoid wheat bran.
	• If you have IBS-C, try eating flaxseeds (see page 42) – up to 4 tablespoons a day for three months (but start with 1 tablespoon a day and build up).
	• If you eat a very-high fibre diet, try reducing this slightly. If you eat a low-fibre diet, then increase it and monitor your symptoms.
	• Use the fibre table to think about what types of fibre are included in your diet, and what may need adjusting.
Think about your fluid intake	Drink 2–3 litres (about 8 glasses) of fluid a day.
Reduce the amount of sugar-free foods you eat	• Reduce your consumption of sugar-free gum, sweets and chocolate.
	• Look out for sorbitol, xylitol and mannitol on food labels.
Give CBT a try	A course of CBT or gut-related hypnotherapy may help.
Try yoga and mindful movement	Regular movement and exercise can help stimulate the bowel. Yoga has been shown to have benefits.
Try probiotics	Try for four weeks and monitor the effects.

3. WHAT IS THE LOW-FODMAP DIET?

Is the low-FODMAP diet better than the first-line advice?

A couple of studies have looked at this. One study in Sweden compared 75 patients with IBS: 38 were given low-FODMAP advice and 37 were given the standard first-line advice for IBS outlined in the previous chapter. People were randomly assigned to these groups for four weeks. The study found very little difference between the two groups at the end of the four weeks: the low-FODMAP group had a 50 per cent reduction in symptoms, while the first-line advice group had a 46 per cent reduction.[30] An analysis of seven randomized controlled trials (good-quality evidence) showed the low-FODMAP diet leads to a one-third reduction in IBS symptoms compared with a control group who were making no changes to their lifestyle.[31] Another study found that, although there was no difference in the amount of people getting a reduction in overall symptoms between a low-FODMAP group and a first-line advice group, there was a difference when you looked at individual symptoms. The low-FODMAP group showed a greater improvement in abdominal pain, bloating, stool consistency and urgency.[32]

The evidence shows us that 50–80 per cent of patients with IBS will get good symptom relief on the low-FODMAP diet in the short term. As I have said, it is not a magic cure, and there are not many long-term research studies (although one study does suggest the benefits continue in 57–74 per cent of patients at 14–16 months).[33]

What does this mean? Well, the first-line advice may work just as well as the more restrictive and complex low-FODMAP diet, so try the simpler stuff out first. Then, combining the two approaches could bring even better results.

There could be some added benefits to the low-FODMAP diet as well. A study showed that it improved quality of life scores, with participants reporting improvements in their body image, as well as in their social and sexual relationships.[34] While that may not be your primary reason for reading this book, it is a fabulous by-product.

How does the low-FODMAP diet work?

As we have learned, FODMAPs are carbohydrates that are poorly absorbed in most people. This is due to our bodies either lacking the enzymes we need to digest them, or them not being well absorbed by the small intestine. People without IBS may still poorly absorb these food particles, but not have IBS symptoms. When these carbohydrates are not properly digested, they enter the colon, with quantities reaching up to 40g (1½oz) a day.[35] In the colon, you will find plant cell walls, resistant starches, bits of protein, and fat. These are broken down by the gut bacteria in a process known as fermentation, and as we've seen, this process releases gas. Some people seem to be more sensitive to this and experience more gut symptoms than others. So while this process is natural and occurs in all of us, if you have a more sensitive gut, then you may experience problems.

Eating certain carbohydrates, including lactose and fructose, has been known to increase IBS symptoms for some time. Other research studies show that giving patients with IBS FODMAPs increases their symptoms, while restricting FODMAPs helps.[36] The low-FODMAP diet therefore works by reducing the amount of FODMAPs eaten, effectively giving the gut a little holiday! Once symptoms are under control, the individual FODMAPs can be reintroduced and tested to find the ideal load for that person. The overall aim is always to reduce symptoms while achieving as diverse a diet as possible and providing all the nutrients the body needs to be healthy.

Q: Are FODMAPs unhealthy?

No. They are found in a range of foods, including fruits, vegetables and wholegrains. There is no need for someone without IBS symptoms to restrict these foods, and in the low-FODMAP process you are aiming to restrict these foods for the shortest time possible.

Why might reducing my consumption of FODMAPs help?

There are a number of reasons why limiting your intake of FODMAPs might have short-term benefits – giving your gut that little 'holiday' I mentioned previously. FODMAPs can affect the digestive system in a variety of ways.

Excess water in the small intestine

Some FODMAPs can increase the amount of water in the small intestine. One study looked at visceral hypersensitivity (when some people react and respond with more sensitivity to gas and bloating than others). Twenty-nine people with IBS and the same number of healthy controls were give a FODMAPs drink containing either fructose, inulin or glucose (not a FODMAP), and then the amount of water in the small bowel and the gas in the colon were measured. Fructose and inulin led to increased symptoms in both groups, with fructose triggering a large increase in water in the small bowel and inulin increasing gas production.[37] This increase in water in the small intestine can cause abdominal pain and bloating in those who are more sensitive. It may also lead to loose stools and diarrhoea.

The production of gas

When there are more carbohydrates in the colon, this leads to more production of gas by the fermenting bacteria. Some people with IBS produce more gas than others, and some seem to be more sensitive to the gas. In the visceral hypersensitivity study above, the amount of gas produced in both groups was similar, but it appeared those with IBS were more sensitive and experienced more abdominal distension. Another study, compared feeding a high-FODMAP diet (50g/1¾oz) per day) to 15 patients with IBS and 15 control patients without IBS. They were then fed a low-FODMAP diet (less than 10g per day). Higher hydrogen was found in the breath of the IBS group compared with the control group on the high-FODMAP diet, and this correlated with increased symptoms.[38] (Please see 'What about breath tests?' on pages 95–6 before rushing out to purchase one.)

Different FODMAPs can lead to different patterns of gas production. Inulin, for example, leads to around double the gas production of other FODMAPs, such as fructose. This is probably due to difference in the absorption of varying FODMAPs and the speed at which they move through the gastrointestinal system.[39] For some people, there is an increased sensitivity to changes in the gut, and they may respond to the changes in levels of gas and water and distension in a stronger way than others. This is not a made-up response, as some people may think, but a very real reaction to what is happening in their body.

Transit time through the gut

FODMAPs could also increase the speed at which matter moves through the colon. If this transit time is reduced, with matter moving through faster, then there is less time for nutrients and FODMAPs to be absorbed over the small intestinal wall. More research needs to be done to look into this.

Balancing the microbiome

We also know that following a low-FODMAP diet changes the gut bacteria and microbes: the levels of specific bacteria in the colon decrease, while the levels of others increase. This makes sense, as following a low-FODMAP diet reduces our consumption of prebiotics, which are the foods feeding the healthy gut bacteria. This may lead to a reduction in healthy gut bacteria (see 'Gut health' on pages 164–7).

Who will the low-FODMAP diet help?

As you read on, you will see how complex this diet is – and how much work it is – so I always check with people if it really is something that they want to do. While there is an element of trial and error to it right now, it could be that in the future microbiome testing or even stool testing will help us know more specifically who can benefit from this diet.

The low-FODMAP diet is considered the only second-line intervention for IBS that has evidence to prove its effectiveness. However, this evidence currently only backs up dietitian-led support, rather than following the diet on your own. This is due to the complexity of the diet. As you read on, you will see how complex this diet is and how much work it is. I always check with people I work with whether it really is something that they want to do.

The low-FODMAP diet can help some people suffering from IBS: the key word here being *some*, not all. As I have said, the low-

FODMAP diet provides a positive response in 50–80 per cent of people with IBS.[40] This means between 20 and 50 per cent of people who follow the low-FODMAP diet will not get better – so how do you know if that is you?

The low-FODMAP diet has been shown to help with some symptoms more than others, and different FODMAPs produce varying symptoms. The research we have shows that symptoms often improve in those suffering from IBS-D and IBS-M, but there is not as much improvement for people suffering from IBS-C. This isn't to say the diet will not help you, of course. Studies have shown improvements in abdominal pain, bloating, flatulence, satisfaction with stool consistency, borborygmi (stomach noises made as food and fluids pass through), urgency and life interference.[41] And it's not just about the physical gut symptoms: let's not forget that the low-FODMAP diet can also improve your overall quality of life.

A number of good-quality randomized controlled trials have now been carried out to look at how well the low-FODMAP diet can help adults with IBS. As always with scientific research, these studies are not all carried out in the same way, and numerous factors play a role in how we should interpret the results, including the size of the samples, whether the groups knew which diet they were on, and how their symptoms were scored. A recent study was carried out over 21 days looking at 30 patients with IBS and 8 healthy controls. The study compared the low-FODMAP diet with a typical diet, with neither group being told which diet they were on, and both groups being given their food. The low-FODMAP diet led to an improvement in gastrointestinal symptoms in 70 per cent of patients, including bloating, pain and wind. Those with IBS-D had fewer toilet trips, and all IBS patients had improved stool consistency.[42] In another blind randomized controlled study, 104 patients with IBS were randomly assigned for 4 weeks to either low-FODMAP advice or a placebo diet that felt healthier than their usual diet and came with the same amount of support as the low-FODMAP group. Those on the low-FODMAP diet had a greater reduction in symptom scores.[43] What is exciting here is that this study did not give people their meals, but instead just gave dietary advice, which is the same level of support you would receive working with a dietitian on the low-FODMAP diet. It suggests that results are possible when people are preparing their own food and managing the diet themselves with the help of a dietitian.

Q: How many times will I need to see my dietitian while on the low-FODMAP diet?

At least twice. You will definitely need to see them at the start of the stage 1 restriction phase, then again at the end of this stage to plan the reintroductions. It is advisable you also see them at the end of stage 2, before you personalize the diet. Depending on your symptoms and overall health, you may need more intensive input.

Other conditions

The low-FODMAP diet has been shown to help with some other conditions too. All of these conditions should be managed by your medical team. Please do not attempt the low-FODMAP diet on your own, as it is highly likely it will need to be adapted for your individual needs.

There is some evidence that people suffering from inflammatory bowel disease (IBD) can respond well to the low-FODMAP diet. Many patients with inactive inflammatory bowel disease (ulcerative colitis or Crohn's disease) have symptoms that are similar to IBS symptoms. A survey showed that around 80 per cent of people suffering from IBD exhibited at least one of the common IBS symptoms.[44] IBS symptoms have been found to be more common in people suffering from inactive Crohn's disease than in those suffering from ulcerative colitis.[45] So can the low-FODMAP diet help? When people diagnosed with inactive IBD who suffer from symptoms of abdominal pain, wind, bloating, diarrhoea or constipation have followed the low-FODMAP diet, around 50 per cent can see an improvement.[46] So it looks pretty promising, but more research is needed to really give clear results.

FODMAPs: the science part

We now know that FODMAPs are types of short-chain carbohydrates (saccharides or sugars) that are poorly absorbed by the digestive system, meaning they pass into the colon where they are fermented, acting as food for the bacteria that live there. For some people, certain FODMAPs can lead to increased fluid or gas, or they may have a heightened sensitivity in the intestines that triggers unwanted bowel symptoms. So let's looks at FODMAPs in a little more detail.

FODMAPs stands for 'Fermentable Oligosaccharides, Disaccharides, Monosaccharides and Polyols'. But what does this actually mean?

Saccharides are sugar units. Monosaccharides are one sugar unit (fructose), disaccharides are two sugar units (lactose), and oligosaccharides are many sugar units (fructans and galacto-oligosaccharides). Polyols are sugars with an alcohol unit attached. Oligosaccharides and sugar alcohols are completely indigestible and cannot be absorbed by the body, but they can be broken down by the gut bacteria to produce gas.

When these FODMAPs arrive in the colon and are fermented by the bacteria there, they produce gases, including butyrate, propionate and acetate, as well as short-chain fatty acids. While this is normal, it leads to stretching of the gut, which can cause abdominal pain. One way to reduce the amount of gas produced is to eat less of these symptom-causing short-chain sugars, but if you did this in the long term, you would be following a very restrictive diet, which is not much fun, limits you socially and could affect your nutritional intake. Therefore, the most practical approach is to work out which are the main culprits. Discover which feed the bacteria the fastest, and reduce these. The FODMAPs have been born! These can be restricted for a few weeks so that symptoms reduce, then gradually reintroduced to find the level each person can tolerate.

All FODMAPs have three common properties:

1. They are poorly absorbed in the intestine. Or, more specifically, the majority of FODMAPs do not get over the intestinal wall for digestion, so they end up in the colon. We all differ in our ability to digest and absorb FODMAPs. We are all slow to digest fructose; some people just don't make much of the enzyme lactase, which is what enables the body to break down lactose; and polyols are an odd shape due to that alcohol unit, so they won't absorb over the intestinal wall. Fructans and galacto-oligosaccharides (GOS) are also poorly absorbed by all of us, although this is worse for some than others. There are three main reasons why this poor digestion happens:

- There may be a lack of enzymes (hydrolases) that break the FODMAPs down and move them over the intestinal wall (or a lack of activity of these enzymes).
- The sugar molecules are too large to pass over the intestinal wall.
- The transport system is just too slow.

2. They are fermented by the bacteria in the colon. This releases gases and by-products that can cause IBS symptoms.

3. They are made up of small chains of sugar molecules joined together. This means digestion and fermentation can happen faster than with larger chains of sugars.[47]

These properties have been shown in research trials. For example, one trial looked at patients who did not have part of their intestine. Instead, they had a stoma bag, which collects the waste products of digestion. A high-FODMAP diet led to there being a higher volume of waste in the stoma bag, showing these sugars were not being well digested.[48]

FODMAPs do not *cause* the gut disorder, but restricting them can help you to reduce your symptoms. While restricting individual FODMAPs is one option, it has limited success. Restricting one individual FODMAP in isolation means other FODMAPs can still be having an impact. Restricting all the FODMAPs at once can seem like a full-on approach, but it does mean that you should see the best results for your symptoms. All FODMAPs can play a role in the symptoms of IBS, but depending on your culture, usual diet and background, you may tend to eat more of one type than another. In the typical Western diet, fructose and fructans are the most common FODMAPs.

A deeper dive into FODMAPs

It is important to note that everyone is different and will have an individual tolerance level for each FODMAP. Remember the ultimate aim of the low-FODMAP diet is to personalize the level of FODMAPs that is right for you, which means you will not have to exclude all the following FODMAPs in the long term.

It's worth remembering that low-FODMAP foods are not *no*-FODMAP foods. All plant-based foods contain some FODMAPs, but you cannot cut out all plant foods, so this is not a black-and-white approach. Everyone responds differently, which is why having a dietitian to talk it through with and support you can be the missing link. Variety is key, so try to eat different low-FODMAP foods throughout your day so you are still eating a range of FODMAPs, just at low levels. For example, even though strawberries are a low-FODMAP food, eating them at each meal may cause symptoms just because you have had so many of them.

So, let's take a closer look at the individual FODMAPs.

Oligosaccharides

These include fructans and galacto-oligosaccharides (GOS). They are found in wheat, rye, lentils, chickpeas, baked beans, onions and garlic.

Fructans

Fructans may be the most common FODMAP to cause symptoms in IBS. They are made up of units of fructose joined together. We all absorb fructans poorly, whether we have IBS or not, as the small intestine does not have the right enzyme to break down the fructose–fructose bonds. Therefore, the fructans pass into the large intestine, where the fermentation process occurs, feeding the beneficial bacteria. As we've seen, this fermentation process can lead to IBS symptoms including gas and bloating. Fructans are found in lots of commonly eaten foods, including bread, some grains, onions and garlic. Smaller amounts can be well tolerated by some people, but others will struggle, with even small amounts triggering IBS symptoms.

Fructans are also found in a variety of other fruit and vegetables (see the 'FODMAPs in fruit and vegetables' table on pages 112–15). These foods are only a problem if they contain more than a certain level of fructans (0.2g per serving for cereals, and 0.3g per serving for other foods). FOS (fructo-oligosaccharides) and oligofructose are additional types of fructans that are often added to particular foods, including certain yogurts and milks, so it is good to keep an eye out for these. Inulin is a lesser-known fructan. This is a starch found in a variety of fruit and vegetables, but it is also a non-digested starch that the gut bacteria can use to improve bowel function. Inulin can be added to foods as a thickening agent, and may be found in yogurts, as well as some prebiotic and probiotic supplements. Always check food labels for inulin, FOS and GOS (see below): they can also be found in things like cereal bars, yogurt-coated snacks, fermented drinks and pre-packed sandwiches.

Foods that only contain a small amount of wheat (such as sauces with wheat-starch thickener) do not need to be cut out, as the level of fructans will be so low. However, foods that contain dried onions and garlic may seem like they would contain low levels, but their fructan content is actually high.

Galacto-oligosaccharides (GOS)

These are chains of galactose sugars with a glucose at the end, and are found in certain vegetables (such as green beans and beetroot) as well as beans, peas, nuts and pulses. There are different types: raffinose and stachyose are the most common. Like fructans, GOS cannot be digested or absorbed by the body as we do not have the enzymes needed to break them down, so they pass to the large intestine for fermentation. The fermentation of GOS increases the growth of beneficial bacteria in our guts. However, in some people with IBS, this process leads to an increase in IBS symptoms. It's common for people to find that restricting GOS helps reduce their symptoms. If you eat a more plant-based diet you are likely to eat more beans and pulses, which could be the cause of some of your IBS symptoms. This doesn't mean you cannot eat these foods – following the low-FODMAP diet will help you find your level of tolerance. We will look at following the low-FODMAP diet when you have a plant-based lifestyle on pages 104–9.

Top tip

Using tinned beans, lentils and pulses rather than fresh or dried makes a difference to their GOS levels, as the FODMAPs leach out into the water in the tin. If you rinse and drain them before eating, therefore, this can reduce the GOS content. Doing this means some people are able to tolerate a medium amount of tinned beans, lentils and pulses.

GOS in foods

High-GOS foods (more than 0.2g GOS per serving)
Kidney beans, cannellini beans, black beans, adzuki beans, baked beans, pinto beans, butter beans, haricot beans, broad beans, chickpeas, lentils

Disaccharides

Disaccharides are formed of two sugar units – glucose and galactose – joined together.

Lactose

Lactose is a disaccharide that occurs naturally in cows' milk, sheep's milk, goats' milk and human milk, plus milk products. It is broken down in the small intestine, by the enzyme lactase, into the individual sugars glucose and galactose, which are then easy for the body to absorb. However, some people do not have enough lactase in their bodies and can only break down a small amount of lactose. The poorly absorbed lactose moves into the small intestine, taking water with it. It then passes undigested into the large intestine, where fermentation occurs. This fermentation causes the symptoms of wind, bloating, stomach cramps and diarrhoea. While lactose intolerance doesn't occur in all people suffering from IBS, it is higher in IBS sufferers. Often people who suffer from it have some idea that lactose is an issue for them before even seeing a dietitian. Lactose intolerance can be genetic, and around 75 per cent of the world's population lose the ability to digest lactose as they age. You are more likely to be lactose intolerant if you are of African, Asian, south European, Hispanic or Mediterranean descent.[49,50] The best way to test for lactose intolerance is to remove lactose from your diet for two weeks, then reintroduce it, gradually increasing your levels to see how much you can tolerate. A lactose-free diet is easily confused with a dairy-free diet, but they are not the same. While lactose is present in some dairy foods, such as milk, the amount present in other dairy foods, such as yogurt, rice pudding and cheeses, varies. There are yogurts and cheese that are almost lactose-free and can be well-tolerated. Most people with lactose intolerance can eat up to 4g lactose per serving without any symptoms. The table overleaf gives you an idea of how much lactose is in common dairy foods.

How much calcium should I have?

Aim for 2–3 portions of calcium-rich foods a day, for example: a glass of fortified milk, a pot of yogurt, 40g (1½oz) cheese, a serving of tofu or tinned fish with bones (sardines, salmon, pilchards).

Lactose in dairy foods

Food/drink	Lactose (in grams)	Low/high lactose
Whole milk (100ml/3½fl oz)	4.4	High, but OK in small amounts
Semi-skimmed milk (100ml/3½fl oz)	4.5	High, but OK in small amounts
Skimmed milk (100ml/3½fl oz)	4.6	High, but OK in small amounts
Evaporated milk (100ml/3½fl oz)	12.1	High
Light evaporated milk (100g/3½oz)	9.8	High
Cottage cheese (40g/1 tbsp)	1.4	Low
Full-fat soft cheese (30g/1 tbsp)	0.5	Low
Feta cheese (40g/1 tbsp)	0.5	Low
Goats' cheese (30g/1 tbsp)	0.25	Low
Hard cheese (Cheddar) (40g/1½oz)	<0.1	Low
Brie and Camembert (40g/1½oz)	<0.1	Low
Low-fat plain yogurt (150g/5½oz)	5–6	OK in moderate amounts
Full-fat plain yogurt (150g/5½oz)	5–6	OK in moderate amounts
Butter/margarine (1 tsp)	0.05	Low

That means while you may not be able to have a glass of milk, having some milk in your cuppa or eating a cake that contains a little can be fine. It is important not to restrict lactose unnecessarily, as this can lead to a low calcium intake, affecting your bone health, and could also lead to a lack of other nutrients, including vitamin D and iodine. Therefore it is important that you only exclude lactose for the minimum time needed, and that the calcium you lose is replaced by fortified plant drinks and substitute yogurts. If you are reducing your lactose intake, take a look at the table on the following pages to see the alternatives you can switch over to. Always check the labels of any substitutes, to make sure calcium has been added at the very least, and ideally iodine and vitamin D as well.

High-lactose foods contain more than 4g lactose per serving, moderate lactose foods contain 1–4g, and low-lactose foods contain less than 1g. It is always key to think about the portion size and not just look at the 'per 100g' amount. This means that foods that are high in lactose can be eaten in small quantities, and that with moderate lactose foods it is important to note the serving sizes you are eating.

High-, moderate- and low-lactose foods

	High-lactose foods (you may need to restrict these on the low-FODMAP diet)	Moderate-lactose foods (limit to one portion per meal)	Low-lactose foods (safe to keep on eating on the low-FODMAP diet)
Milk and milk products	• all types of cows', goats' and sheep's milk • cows' milk powder • evaporated milk • condensed milk • soy milk from soy beans	• a dash of cows' milk in tea/coffee • 15ml (1 tbsp) kefir • <30ml (1fl oz) oat milk drink in UK* • 50ml (2fl oz) sweetened soy milk drink • <70g (2½oz) buttermilk • 120ml (4fl oz) unsweetened soy milk (from soy beans) • <125ml (4fl oz) coconut milk drink • 120ml (4fl oz) hemp milk drink • 200ml (7fl oz) rice milk drink • 120ml (4fl oz) tinned coconut milk	• lactose-free milk • nut milk drink (hazelnut, macadamia and almond) – choose fortified versions • unsweetened quinoa milk • 19g (¾oz) butter • coconut milk powder • soy milk from soy protein • coconut cream

	High-lactose foods (you may need to restrict these on the low-FODMAP diet)	Moderate-lactose foods (limit to one portion per meal)	Low-lactose foods (safe to keep on eating on the low-FODMAP diet)
Desserts	Cows' milk products: • ice cream • rice pudding and milky desserts • custard made with cows' milk	• 1 scoop (85g/3oz) cows' milk ice cream • 2 tbsp (75g/2¾oz) custard • 80g (2¾oz) soured cream • double cream • 30g (1oz) milk/white chocolate	• soy custard • plain soy ice cream • dark chocolate • crème fraîche • 60g (2¼oz) whipped cream • lactose-free ice cream
Yogurt	• cows', sheep's and goats' milk yogurts • fromage frais	• 60g (2¼oz) natural yogurt • 93g (c.3⅓oz) plain Greek yogurt • soy yogurt (check flavours) • 80g (2¾oz) vanilla yogurt	• lactose-free strawberry and raspberry yogurt • coconut yogurt (check the label for other FODMAPs)

	High-lactose foods (you may need to restrict these on the low-FODMAP diet)	Moderate-lactose foods (limit to one portion per meal)	Low-lactose foods (safe to keep on eating on the low-FODMAP diet)
Cheese	• processed cheese and cheese slices • garlic and herb cheeses • reduced-fat Cheddar	Up to 40g (1½oz) of: • cottage cheese • cream cheese • halloumi • low-fat soft cheese • quark • ricotta • small soft cheese triangles (1 triangle)	40g (1½oz) most hard cheese and ripened cheese: • blue cheese • Brie • Camembert • Cheddar • Edam • Emmental • feta • goats' cheese • Gorgonzola • Gouda • Gruyère • mozzarella • paneer • Parmesan • Pecorino • raclette • soy cheese • Stilton • Swiss cheese

*This may differ between individual countries.

Monosaccharides

Fructose

Commonly known as the sugar in fruit, high-fructose foods include mangos, apples, pears, asparagus, sugar snap peas, figs, honey, dried fruit and fruit juice. Fructose is only poorly absorbed in some people, and leads to there being excess water in the small intestine. While it is not certain that you will have to restrict high-fructose foods, if you are not sure, it makes sense to restrict them. Some people will be totally fine with fructose. So how do you know?

It can be useful to spend some time looking at the foods that are high in fructose and thinking about whether any of these foods appear to cause symptoms for you. In some foods, fructose is found with glucose: think of the two as best friends who cross over the small intestine wall using transporter trucks. Now, fructose on its own can move over the small intestine wall using the transport molecule GLUT-5. This is not a very efficient system, and there aren't many GLUT-5 transporters around, so when there is a lot of fructose about, a traffic jam builds up. This is known as fructose malabsorption, and it causes gut symptoms (commonly diarrhoea, but it can cause any of the IBS symptoms mentioned earlier).

Some people are better equipped to deal with fructose than others. If you have fructose malabsorption, it doesn't mean you need to avoid fruit altogether. Instead, you need to eat fructose together with glucose. With glucose around, fructose is happier, as now another transporter (GLUT-2) can be used and this has more capacity to transport the sugars over the intestinal wall. Happier tummy ensues.

Did you know that fructose + glucose = sucrose? The body deals better with sucrose than fructose on its own. The amount of free fructose (not connected to glucose) we can digest varies from person to person: up to half the population are unable to absorb a load of 25g, and the average daily intake of fructose varies from 11–54g a day.[51] Some foods can be problematic if you have fructose malabsorption.[52] This may mean you need to eat less of certain fruits, such as mango (my favourite). Breath testing can be done to measure your responses (see pages 95–6), but you can also use the table on the following pages to help you avoid all foods with extra fructose, and aim to eat foods where glucose and fructose are in balance instead. This can sound confusing, and that's where your dietitian comes in – to help you work out which fruits are right for you.

Fructose in foods

	Excess fructose (eat less or avoid altogether)	Low fructose or more glucose than fructose (safe to eat)
Fruit	• apples • cherries • figs • mangos • pears • watermelon • apple/pear fruit juice	In small quantities: • apricots • avocados • bananas • blackberries • blueberries • cantaloupe melon • cranberries • grapefruit • grapes • honeydew melon • jackfruit • kiwifruit • lemons • limes • nectarines • oranges • papayas • passion fruit • peaches • pineapples • plums • raspberries • rhubarb • strawberries • tangerines • tomatoes

	Excess fructose (eat less or avoid altogether)	Low fructose or more glucose than fructose (safe to eat)
Vegetables	• asparagus • artichokes (Jersulaem) • broccoli stalks • sugar snap peas	all other low-FODMAP vegetables (see page 118)
Sugars and spreads	• agave • fructose • fruit juice concentrate • high-fructose corn syrup • honey • ketchup • pickles	In moderate amounts: • brown sugar • cane sugar • caster sugar • coconut sugar • glucose • granulated sugar • jam and marmalade (limit to 100% fruit spreads) • maple syrup • molasses • nut butters (not cashew) • palm sugar • rice syrup • sucrose • yeast extract (Marmite)

A simple approach to fructose

The gut is easily overloaded by fructose. An easier way to deal with this is to only eat one portion of fruit per meal/snack, and spread it out throughout the day, leaving a minimum of two hours between portions.

Eat one of the below at a meal/snack, then wait at least two hours before eating another portion:

- 1 banana
- 1 orange
- 2 kiwifruit
- 2 satsumas
- 1 slice of melon or pineapple
- 100ml (3½fl oz) fruit juice (not apple or pear) – you can dilute this with water for a longer drink
- 1 small handful of berries or grapes
- 20g (¾oz) dried fruit
- 3 tablespoons tomato purée or fruit chutney

Polyols

Polyols, or sugar alcohols, are often used as artificial sweeteners or water-binding agents. They include the '-ols' : sorbitol (E420), mannitol (E421), maltitol (E965), xylitol (E967), polydextrose (E1200) and isomalt (E953). They occur in some fruit and vegetables, including cauliflower, mushrooms, pears and apples, as shown in the table on the following pages. Sugar-free gum, chocolate and sweets can contain sorbitol or xylitol, so do check the labels. Foods containing more than 0.5g polyols per serving can trigger IBS symptoms.

Polyols in foods

	High in polyols	Moderate polyols	Low in polyols
Fruit	• apples • apricots • blackberries • nectarines • peaches • plums • prunes • watermelon	• ¼ avocado • 3 cherries • 5 lychees	• bananas • blueberries • cantaloupe melon • cranberries • grapefruit • grapes • honeydew melon • kiwifruit • lemons • limes • mangos • oranges • papayas • passion fruit • pineapple • raspberries • rhubarb • strawberries • tangerines

	High in polyols	Moderate polyols	Low in polyols
Vegetables	• cauliflower • mangetout • mushrooms • peas	• 1 stalk celery • 7 pods mangetout • 100g (3½oz) sweet potato	all other low-FODMAP vegetables
Sugar-free foods	• chewing gum, mints and sweets made with artificial sweeteners (isomalt, maltitol, mannitol, polydextrose, sorbitol, xylitol)		• chewing gum made with sugar/sucrose • sugar-sweetened sweets and mints
Additives	• isomalt • maltitol • mannitol • polydextrose • sorbitol • xylitol		• aspartame • saccharine • stevia

How are FODMAPs tested?

The Monash University team test for FODMAPs under laboratory conditions. They take a range of samples of the food to find the average FODMAP content. There are FODMAP cut-off points used to determine if a food is high, medium or low in FODMAPs, which has led to the traffic light system of red (high), amber (moderate) and green (low). As this is still pretty new, not all foods have been tested, and there can be differences between products from one country to another due to the ingredients used. Products are constantly being reformulated so foods have to be retested, which takes time.

While the internet is a wonderful place in many ways, it is also full of conflicting information. Exercise caution when looking at lists of low-FODMAP foods, unless they have come from your dietitian. King's College London produce booklets that are very useful: while you cannot buy these booklets yourself, your dietitian may give you one. You might also want to explore apps, such as the Monash University FODMAP Diet app or the FODMAP by FM app (see Resources, pages 247–8). Some apps have a barcode system that allows you to scan foods to check them. Your dietitian should also be able to help you: do use their knowledge. If you are unsure about a certain food, it is always worth checking. Remember: it is the total amount of FODMAPs ingested that is the key factor.

The FODMAP traffic lights

RED = High-FODMAP content – do not eat on the restriction stage of the diet.

AMBER = Moderate-FODMAP content – you can eat small amounts of these foods on the restriction stage of the diet.

GREEN = Low-FODMAP content – you can eat these foods on the restriction stage of the diet.

4. STAGE 1: THE RESTRICTION STAGE

S o, now you have explored the first-line advice, read about how the diet works, and where the FODMAPs are found, it's time to make a start.

Always keep your GP up to date and chat to them about progressing to the next stage. You should also ask them for advice on where to access dietitian support (see pages 86–7).

While the normal route with the low-FODMAP diet is to restrict all FODMAPs for four to eight weeks, there is a simplified version that can be used too. If you are someone for whom a restrictive diet is not helpful, then you can focus on only restricting the main high-FODMAP foods, along with any suspected trigger foods. This could be useful if you have previously suffered from an eating disorder, or if you have a very limited intake of foods to begin with. If you have an active eating disorder, then now is not the right time to be following the low-FODMAP diet. It's important for you to focus on your recovery first.

It is easier to follow this first stage of the diet if you do not eat out too frequently, and if you are able to cook most of your meals from scratch. However, that is not always possible and food is a huge part of our social lives too! There are lots of recipes out there (including the ones in this book) to help you out so please do use them. Check out the Resources (pages 247–52) for more options.

Before you begin

Find a dietitian

This is a crucial step before you get started. You can ask your GP to refer you to a dietitian (there may be a waiting list for this, but you can use the time to read and prepare). Alternatively, see the Resources section (pages 247–52) if you are thinking about looking for a private dietitian. The support you access could be in person or virtual. Some GPs may suggest you simply follow Google and go it alone, which I would strongly dissuade you from. The low-FODMAP diet was designed to be followed with specialist support, and having that support in place really can make all the difference.[53] It may seem easy to just cut out certain foods and think you have eliminated all FODMAPs, but trust me, FODMAPs are sneaky! Most specialist dietitians will tell you how often we come across people who have tried this diet on their own without success, because they were actually still eating FODMAPs without realizing it. It can be a bit like looking for that needle in the haystack. There are also other factors to consider, such as smaller amounts of FODMAPs stacking up, the nutritional adequacy of your diet and practical consideration of how this will really work with your lifestyle.

Always check that the dietitian you are working with knows about the low-FODMAP diet. Ideally, you will work with someone who has had specialist training in this area. It is especially important that older adults and children work closely with a dietitian, and they may also find it better to use the simplified approach outlined on page 85.

Why can't I just follow the low-FODMAP diet on my own?
If your car was broken, would you try to fix it yourself? Probably not. A trusted mechanic is always going to be the best option. The same applies here: dietitians are the trusted experts. Here's why it's important to consult a dietitian before attempting this diet.

- FODMAPs can be hidden in unexpected places. They have tricky names and are easy to miss. Sometimes you can think you have cut out all FODMAPs, but there are still a few sneaky ones there. An expert eye can help you find them.
- The restriction stage of this diet involves cutting out a lot of your normal foods. It is so important that you replace these foods with appropriate alternatives that still meet your nutritional needs. Having a dietitian advise you on how to individualize your FODMAP diet while still meeting your nutritional needs is paramount.
- The reintroduction and personalization stages of the low-FODMAP diet also require good planning and motivation. A professional who can keep you on track and reassure you can be such a help here.

- Following this diet without professional support is less likely to be effective. Trust me: I've met plenty of people who have attempted the diet on their own, who then realized the importance of having professional support. The evidence we have shows beneficial results *when the diet is followed with dietitian support*. There isn't evidence to show it being effective without this level of specialist support.[54]

- If you suffer from another medical condition as well as IBS, you will need to work closely with your dietitian to see if there are any special considerations you need to take into account. For example, you may need to make some changes to your medications if you have diabetes; if you have other food allergies, these will need to be taken into account; and there can be times in your life when it is just not a good idea to start the low-FODMAP diet. A dietitian can help you make sure you're making the right choices for you.

Preparing to meet your dietitian

Before you meet with your dietitian, it can be helpful to gather together a folder of useful information so you can make the most of your session. Do not feel worried about talking about your bowels and poo! For dietitians, this is all part of the job and very normal.

Here are some useful things you can do to prepare:

- Keep a diary for one to three weeks showing your normal eating, drinking and exercise habits.
- Track your bowel habits, IBS symptoms, sleep and stress levels for three weeks. You can use an app, such as Bowelle, or an IBS tracker (see Resources, page 247–52).

- Try out meditation or yoga and note any changes these make to your IBS symptoms.
- Collate the results of any recent blood or breath tests (see pages 11 and 95–6).
- Think about how often you eat out and the main places you go.

Plan, plan and plan again!

Stock up your cupboards with FODMAP-friendly foods (some handy hints are given in the box on page 90). While the elimination phase is only four to eight weeks, you also need to restrict those FODMAPs in stage 2, so get ready to change how you eat for a minimum of three months.

Write out your usual meal plan for four weeks. If you have kept a food diary, this will make it nice and easy. Now you can play 'hunt the FODMAPs' and work out which foods you need to substitute. The aim is to end up with a range of tasty and nutritious breakfasts, lunches, dinners and snacks that are low in FODMAPs. This is not a weight-loss plan, so include all your usual extras and the foods that bring you pleasure. Then check this with your dietitian.

Think about any travel plans you have coming up: you may want to start the elimination phase *after* any holidays or work trips you have planned. If you travel regularly for work, plan what you will need to take with you and look at menus to get an idea of what you will be able to order. For more tips on eating out, see pages 135–6.

Stocking up on FODMAP-friendly foods

Stock up on foods that will add plenty of flavour to your meals:

• asafoetida – a good substitute for onion and garlic

• plenty of herbs and spices – basil, cardamom, chilli (powder and flakes), chives, cinnamon, fresh and ground coriander, fennel seeds, fresh and ground ginger, mustard, nutmeg, paprika, parsley, rosemary, thyme, turmeric

• lemon juice

• soy sauce*, oyster sauce*, coconut milk*, tamarind paste, fish sauce, Worcestershire sauce, wasabi powder, nutritional yeast

• nuts and seeds (not cashews and pistachios)

For more ideas, see 'Cooking tips' on pages 132–3.

*Please check suitable amounts on the Monash University FODMAP Diet app as these ingredients contain some FODMAPs.

Q: *Should I avoid all FODMAPs?*

This is something to discuss with your dietitian. If you have previously tested your tolerance for lactose and know it is not a trigger for you, or if know you can absorb fructose, you may not need to restrict those FODMAPs. It is normal to restrict the rest.

Stacking and serving sizes

As you look at the tables in this chapter, you will see that there are some foods that contain moderate levels of FODMAPs. These are important foods, as they add variety and nutrition to your diet, but it is vital to focus on the serving sizes. These foods are only moderate in FODMAPs if you eat that serving size or less. If you eat too many of the moderate-FODMAP foods in one day or one meal, it can overload your system, increasing your symptoms. Keep a detailed food diary of what you eat, along with the portion sizes. Highlight any moderate-FODMAP foods you have eaten, and note any symptoms you have. Everyone has different thresholds for these FODMAPs, so take a look through your diary and see what patterns you find. You may find you can only tolerate one moderate-FODMAP food per meal, or you may be OK with a couple. FODMAPs are like building blocks: they all add up over the day. FODMAPs can also be affected by things like pickling, sprouting and the way a food is processed. Interestingly, among the foods that have been tested so far, pickling and sprouting seem to reduce the FODMAP content of foods, but not everything has been tested, so always bear in mind how your food is processed and check it on the food lists/apps. Remember: low-FODMAP does not mean no FODMAPs, and eating lots of low- or moderate-FODMAP foods can mean the FODMAPs you are eating pile up. Spread out that fruit, and eat different colours and types of foods throughout the day to minimize any symptoms. Remember that this is a trial-and-error approach. Sometimes it will go wrong, and that's OK: treat it as a learning moment.

Multiple types of the different FODMAP groups are usually present in one meal, and sometimes multiple FODMAPs are found in one food. This can make it hard to work out where your symptoms are coming from.

How FODMAPs can add up over the day, triggering symptoms

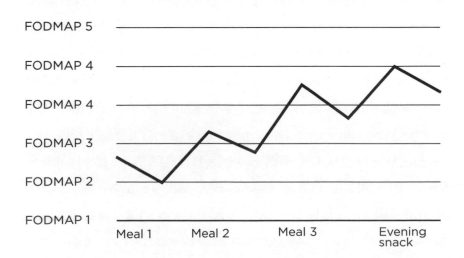

Stick with the monitoring and food diary. It is not just the individual FODMAPs that can be the issue, but the way these FODMAPS can stack up throughout the day. This is why it is key to look at your diet as a whole, and not just focus on the individual foods eaten. Another added complication is that the FODMAP content of foods can vary from country to country, and is affected by ripeness, storage and seasonal variations. Foods are also constantly being retested for their FODMAP content, which can explain why some websites will give different answers. Staying up to date is really important, so although the information and food lists in this book are a guide, always look to your dietitian and use the Monash University FODMAP Diet app or the updated FODMAP by FM app for queries.

What to look out for on food labels

Always check food labels, even if it seems like the food is likely to be low in FODMAPs. Gluten-free foods can use apple juice as a sweetener, or may include chickpea flour (gram flour) as an ingredient, while garlic and onion are used in many products.

Do think about the portion sizes you eat, too, as FODMAPs will vary if you have a larger portion of a food than the portion given on the label.

If you are unsure, either consult one of the FODMAP apps or ask your dietitian.

Key ingredients to look out for on food labels

If a label lists:	It contains:
• agave • dried fruit • fructose • fruit juice • fruit juice concentrate • fruit sugar • honey • high-fructose corn syrup	Fructose
• erythritol • isomalt • mannitol • sorbitol • xylitol	Polyols
• chicory, chicory root • flavour, flavouring, natural flavour (this can mean onion/garlic) • fructo-oligosaccharide (FOS) • garlic, garlic salt, garlic powder, garlic extract • inulin • onion, onion salt, onion powder, onion extract • rye • wheat	Fructans

*Q: Can I have a cheat day or
do I need to be super strict?*

*While the restriction stage is hard, it is important to try and stick to
it as well as you can in order to get those symptoms under control.
We are aiming to clean out FODMAPs from the system and give it
a rest. So if you keep eating small amounts, you may not see the full
benefits. Having said that, life happens and a one-off slip in a meal
shouldn't send you back to day one.*

What about breath tests?

There are breath tests available that measure the
hydrogen in your breath after consuming a test dose
of sugars: this is thought to be a way to tell if you are
sensitive to certain FODMAPs. These tests are not
always easy to get done and are not available in all
areas due to reservations about their accuracy.

The science behind the tests is that, as gut bacteria
ferment foods, they release hydrogen, as well as some
methane. Some of this hydrogen is absorbed into the
bloodstream and makes its way out of the body via
the lungs, leading to hydrogen in the breath. The only
reason you would have hydrogen in your breath is due
to those gut bacteria fermenting foods, which would
suggest you have an intolerance. The test is simple:

you need to limit your FODMAP and fibre intake for 24 hours, then fast for several hours before the test. You then take a solution of fructose or lactose, before breathing into a machine at intervals over the course of 2–3 hours. Some websites claim that these tests will show if you are intolerant to lactose/fructose. While that would make life much easier, and could make the diet less restrictive, there are issues.

Firstly, you have to consume a dose of the sugar that is larger than you would normally eat, giving an exaggerated result. A review in 2016 found that people suffering from IBS had the same results from these tests as those who didn't, suggesting the tests do not accurately detect whether you suffer from IBS symptoms after eating these FODMAPs. If you do not have symptoms, you don't need to stop eating these sugars. People were also found to get different results on different days. The final confirmation that these tests are not accurate enough was that 20–25 per cent of IBS sufferers who had a negative breath test were found to have IBS symptoms when eating foods with fructose/lactose in them. For these reasons, breath tests are not widely used. If you do have a breath test done, it is best to then confirm your result by excluding the FODMAP group and later reintroducing it as a food challenge.

What can I eat?

The start of the elimination phase can feel very overwhelming: suddenly you need to read all the food labels, check all your meals and alter recipes, and it can feel like there's nothing you're allowed to eat. Don't despair! I'm going to talk you through what you *can* eat. There are also plenty of recipes in this book, and many other good low-FODMAP recipe books available. Some are listed in the Resources section (see page 251).

The first step is to make sure that each meal contains a balance of protein, carbohydrate, fruit/veg and fats/dairy. Focusing on balanced meals can help you ensure you meet your nutritional needs. So, let's think through the food groups.

Food groups and servings

	Servings per day	Examples for low-FODMAP diet
Fruit	Minimum of 2, maximum of 5	2 kiwifruit 2 satsumas 1 large handful of strawberries
Vegetables	5–7 portions a day	80g (2¾oz/ 1 handful) carrots, tomatoes, peppers or other low-FODMAP vegetables

	Servings per day	Examples for low-FODMAP diet
Dairy/calcium foods	3–4 portions a day	150ml (¼ pint) low-lactose milk 150g (5½oz) low-lactose yogurt 40g (1½oz) low-lactose cheese (see the table on page 74 for examples of these)
Fats and oils	Limit to 1–2 a day	1 tablespoon oil, butter or margarine
Protein foods	2–3 portions	80–100g (2¾–3½oz) meat 100–125g (3½–4½oz) fish 2 eggs 170–200g (6–7oz) tofu 25g (1oz) nuts or seeds
Carbohydrate foods	At least 4	1 slice of gluten-free bread 75–100g (2¾–3½oz) cooked grains 30g (1oz) oats 30g (1oz) low-FODMAP breakfast cereal

Carbohydrates

This can be seen as the tricky part for some people, as if you cut out wheat, what are you going to eat? As someone who has been wheat-free for medical reasons for years, I can tell you there are lots of options!

You need to avoid wheat, rye and barley. This cuts out standard bread, pasta, cakes and biscuits. It is important to check the labels of any gluten-free products: don't assume that being gluten-free makes them low in FODMAPs. They can still include onion, garlic and fruit juice.

Once you have eliminated wheat for a few weeks, you may find you are able to tolerate 100 per cent spelt sourdough bread.

Super spelt sourdough

Although spelt is an ancestor of wheat, spelt flour is lower in FODMAPs. The fermentation process that takes place when making sourdough bread reduces the FODMAP content further, making 100 per cent spelt sourdough bread suitable for those on the low-FODMAP diet.

Carbohydrates on the low-FODMAP diet

	Wheat versions to avoid	Alternatives
Bread	• all wheat breads and bread products (pitta, bagels, rolls, pancakes, muffins, pastries, wraps, pizza base, soda bread) • chapatti, naan, flatbread or roti • rye, barley and pumpernickel bread • wheat or rye sourdough	• bread made using oats, quinoa, maize, millet, buckwheat, cornmeal, rice, potato, tapioca flour • dosa, plain • 100% spelt sourdough bread • wheat-free or gluten-free breads (remember to check the label for apple juice or onion/garlic) • wonton wrapper

	Wheat versions to avoid	Alternatives
Pasta and grains	• amaranth • bulgur wheat • couscous • egg and udon noodles • farro • freekeh • gnocchi (unless it uses wheat-free flour) • pearl barley • semolina • wheat, spelt, red lentil and pea pasta	• chickpea pasta (up to 100g/3½oz cooked weight) • gluten-free couscous (made from maize flour) • gluten-free gnocchi • gluten-free pasta • kelp noodles • polenta • quinoa • quinoa pasta • rice • rice noodles/pasta • soba noodles • 100% spelt sourdough pasta
Breakfast cereals	• bran cereal • spelt flakes • wheat cereal • wheat flakes	• buckwheat groats • cornflakes • oats, porridge and oat flakes, oat biscuits, make-your-own muesli • quinoa and rice flakes • rice cereals

	Wheat versions to avoid	Alternatives
Crackers	• All crackers containing wheat, rye and barley (eg cream crackers, cheese biscuits, digestive crackers, rye crispbread, spelt crackers)	• 100% buckwheat crackers • corn cakes • gluten-free crackers • oatcakes • rice cakes and rice crackers
Cakes and biscuits	All cakes and biscuits made with wheat flour	• almond and polenta cakes • flourless cakes • gluten-free cakes/ biscuits • oat biscuits and flapjacks (check label for flour)
Pastry and bread-crumbs	• all pastry made with wheat flour • all wheat breadcrumbs	• crushed cornflakes, puffed rice cereal or oats instead of breadcrumbs • gluten-free pastry mixes/ready to roll
Other cereal products and flours	• amaranth, barley, coconut, rye, spelt flour • chickpea/gram flour • wheat flours	• arrowroot • buckwheat flour • chestnut flour • corn/maize • millet • polenta • potato flour • quinoa • rice • sorghum • tapioca • teff flour

Fats and oils

As a general rule, none of these contain FODMAPs. Do, however, beware of flavoured oils or oils with garlic cloves in the bottle. You can use garlic-infused oil (see pages 132–3) as long as you do not consume or cook with the garlic cloves.

Protein

Most animal protein sources are low in FODMAPs. You want to be eating protein two to three times a day. It is important to eat enough protein for your body to renew and repair cells, and to help look after your nervous system, immune system, enzyme reactions, muscles and more. You can see how vital this is. All plain meat, fish, chicken and eggs are FODMAP-free and safe to eat: just be careful with any sauces, stock cubes, onions and garlic that you may add as you cook them, as well as anything that is breaded or battered.

The low-FODMAP diet for vegetarians and vegans

Beans and pulses

If you are vegetarian or vegan, you may find it concerning that legumes, beans and pulses need to be restricted, as you probably use these as one of your main protein sources. However, they contain FODMAPs. It is totally possible to follow the restriction phase of the low-FODMAP diet if you have a plant-based lifestyle, but you will need to a little more creative. Small amounts of beans and pulses are allowed, but as these are moderate-FODMAP foods, they do stack up, meaning it is best to vary your protein sources over your day and week. For example, you could have 2 tablespoons of chickpeas with your lunch, and then tofu with dinner. Rinsing and draining tinned varieties of beans and lentils will help keep their FODMAP content lower. Firm tofu (not silken), miso and tempeh are made from soybeans, which are high in FODMAPs, but the fermentation and processing they undergo reduces their FODMAP content (silken tofu is not processed in the same way, and remains high in FODMAPs). Do be sure to check the labels for any added flavourings, like onions and garlic. Seitan is made from wheat protein and is therefore not suitable.

Soy

Some soy dairy replacement products are low in FODMAPs and make good protein sources, but not all of them. Soy milks made from soy bean extract or soy protein are suitable, but the whole soy bean is high in the FODMAPs raffinose and stachyose (types of galacto-oligosaccharides) and not suitable, so again it is important to check the label. Another thing to be aware of is that soy flour contains FODMAPs, so it is not suitable, but it is sometimes used in gluten-free foods. Again, this is why reading the label or using a good FODMAP food list is so important. You may need to work with your dietitian to establish your tolerance to soy products, as some people are better with them than others. Most nuts and seeds are suitable if you stick to a small handful (less than 25g): this includes some nut butters and nut alternatives to milk.

Other protein options

Other ways to meet your protein needs in the restriction stage include using grains: quinoa, buckwheat, oats and even rice will provide some protein. Choose breakfast cereals and breads made from quinoa, buckwheat or chia for a protein boost. Low-lactose dairy can also help with protein: I've included more about this the dairy section (see pages 109–10). Soy mince or mycoprotein can be a good protein source, and pea protein powder can be added as a top-up if you are concerned about not getting enough. As always, check the labels of all products for FODMAPs, as they do creep in when you least expect them.

FODMAPs in plant-based proteins

High-FODMAP	Moderate-FODMAP	Low-FODMAP
• large amounts (more than in the moderate column) of lentils, beans, baked beans and pulses • soy beans • pistachios • cashews • flavoured/ marinated protein labels need to be checked • textured vegetable protein (TVP)	• 45g (1¾oz) black beans • 3 tbsp (60g/2¼oz) butter beans • 200g (7oz) frozen edamame beans • 3 tbsp (84g/c.3oz) tinned chickpeas (rinsed and drained) • 1 tbsp (46g/c.1¾oz) boiled red or green lentils	• 45g (1¾oz) tinned pinto beans (rinsed and drained) • 8g (c.¼oz) spirulina • tempeh • firm tofu (not silken) • 95g (3⅓oz) mung beans, sprouted • 2–3 tbsp (25g/1oz) nuts and seeds (max. 10 almonds and hazelnuts) • 2 tbsp nut butter • 2 tbsp (46g/c.1¾oz) tinned lentils (rinsed and drained) • 75g (2¾oz) mycoprotein

If you are vegetarian, vegan or plant-based, take a look at the protein chart on pages 107–8 and think about how you can meet your protein needs over a week using a range of protein sources. Aim for around 50g (1¾oz) protein a day, which you can easily meet if you have around 20g (¾oz) protein at each main meal. No one wants to eat the same meals every day, and eating a variety of foods helps you meet all your micronutrient needs, too.

Plant-based protein sources

20g protein	10g protein	5g protein	2.5g protein
100g (3½oz) tempeh	150–200g (5½–7oz) soya yogurt	150ml (¼ pint) soya milk	45g (1¾oz) edamame (not soy) beans
80g (2¾oz) tofu	4 oatcakes	150g (5½oz) cooked wheat-free pasta	2 tbsp (44g/c.1¾oz) chickpeas (either tinned or dried and cooked)
25–30g (1oz) seitan (you can meet your day's protein needs in a 100g/3½oz serving)	100g (3½oz) mycoprotein (not TVP)	1 large baked potato	2 tbsp (44g/c.1¾oz) tinned lentils or chana dhal
	2 eggs	25g (1oz) max. sunflower, chia, pumpkin or other seeds	2 slices of wheat-free bread
	40g (1½oz) Cheddar	<25g (1oz) walnuts	10 almonds
	2 tbsp nut butter	60g (2¼oz) wheat-free cereal flakes	95g (3⅓oz) mung beans, sprouted
		100g (3½oz) cooked quinoa	
		140g (5oz) cooked rice	
		70g (2½oz) cooked couscous	

20g protein	10g protein	5g protein	2.5g protein
		45g (1¾oz) porridge oats	
		60g (2¼oz) wheat-free cereal flakes	

Plant-based protein ideas

- Nibble on nuts and seeds between meals, or add them as a topping to cereal or yogurt – but limit your portion to less than 25g (1oz), or 10 nuts for almonds and hazelnuts.

- Try to eat a wide variety of grains: quinoa, and couscous are good examples.

- Get to grips with different tofu, tempeh and seitan recipes. You can use them to make an alternative to scrambled eggs, or use them in a stir-fry or even in a smoothie.

- Choose breakfast cereals and breads made with buckwheat, quinoa or chia.

- If you eat eggs, include these throughout the week.

Plant-based meal ideas with protein

Breakfast

- 60g (2¼oz) wheat-free flakes with 150ml (¼ pint) milk, 25g (1oz) seeds and strawberries (12.5g protein)
- Scrambled firm tofu on 2 slices of wheat-free bread with cooked peppers and spinach (22.5g protein)

Lunch

- 4 oatcakes with 40g (1½oz) Cheddar, tomatoes, raw carrot and olives (20g protein)
- 2 boiled eggs in an egg-mayo sandwich (wheat-free bread) with low-FODMAP vegetables and 150g (5½oz) plant alternative to yogurt (22.5g protein)

Dinner

- 100g (3½oz) mycoprotein made into a chilli, served with rice and 44g (c.1¾oz/2 tablespoons) tinned lentils (2.5g protein)
- 150g (5½oz) wheat-free pasta with tomato sauce (no onion/garlic), 25g (1oz) sunflower seeds mixed into the sauce (5g protein), 40g (1½oz) Cheddar grated on top (20g protein) and topped with a handful of mung bean sprouts

Dairy

If you are not restricting lactose, then it is fine to keep eating dairy, but do avoid cheeses made with onions and garlic. Tasty, but sadly not suitable right now. If you are not eating lactose, then there are actually still a lot of dairy foods you can eat, as many cheeses are low in lactose, and you can still eat small amounts of lactose. Take a look at the 'Lactose in dairy foods' table on page 70 and the 'High-, moderate- and low-lactose foods' table on pages 72–4. Choose a lactose-free milk or a nut-based alternative to milk (such as almond, hazelnut or macadamia); find a low-FODMAP yogurt you like; and remember most cheese is allowed. It is important to check your milk alternative is fortified with calcium and preferably also with iodine. A top tip is to make sure you shake the milk before you use it, as the calcium can sink to the bottom in some brands.

Fruit and vegetables

All plant foods contain FODMAPs, so this can feel like a tricky food group to navigate, but it is still important to keep eating them. Aim to eat a variety of colours and types of fruit and veggies from the low-FODMAP group throughout your day and week. How about seeing this as a time to try some new foods and experiment with new meals? It's an adventure! The main FODMAPs present are excess fructose and sorbitol in fruit, and mannitol and fructans in vegetables. Boiling rather than roasting butternut squash, spaghetti squash and sweet potatoes will help lower the FODMAP content of these moderate-FODMAP foods. Choose pickled rather than fresh onions and beetroot, as these may be better tolerated. Some sprouted seeds and beans may also be suitable: you can try these with caution, as many have not yet been tested. Note that sprouted chickpeas are high in FODMAPs, but bean sprouts are low in FODMAPs.

Drinks

Most drinks are suitable on the low-FODMAP diet. However, you need to be careful with alcohol, juices, smoothies and protein shakes. Many alcoholic drinks are low in FODMAPs, but they can still trigger symptoms for some people, so stick to no more than one or two units a day of alcohol and consume it with food. Also, remember that caffeine can be a trigger for symptoms, so either choose caffeine-free drinks or keep your caffeine to sensible levels (three cups of coffee a day, or three to four cups of tea). It is important to stay hydrated to aid your bowels, so aim for six to eight glasses of water a day

Most diet soft drinks are suitable, but do check which sweetener has been added using the 'Key ingredients to look out for on food labels' table on page 94. Nut and lactose-free milk can be enjoyed throughout the day, or added to tea and coffee. Fruit juice can be suitable in small amounts: just stay away from apple and pear juice. Choose 100ml (3½fl oz) orange, cranberry, pineapple or tomato juice, and dilute with water to make it go further. Squash and cordials can be fine, but check the labels once again.

FODMAPs in fruit and vegetables

Food	High in FODMAPs	Moderate levels of FODMAPs	
Fruit	• apples • apricots • bananas (ripe) • blackberries • cherries • cranberries, dried • currants • dates • figs • goji berries, dried • mangos • nectarines • peaches • pears • persimmons • plums • prunes • watermelon	• ¼ avocado • ½ small ripe banana (45g/1¾oz) • 50g (1¾oz) blueberries • 96g (c.3⅓oz) whole coconut • 4 lychees • 1 tbsp raisins • 35 raspberries • 2 tsp (7g/¼oz) sultanas	

Low in FODMAPs	
• bananas (firm)	• oranges
• clementines	• papayas
• 30g (1oz) shredded dried coconut	• passion fruit
• grapefruit	• pineapples
• grapes	• plantains
• guava	• rhubarb
• jackfruit	• strawberries
• kiwifruit	• tangerines
• kumquats	
• lemons	
• limes	
• mandarins	
• <100g (3½oz) melons (cantaloupe and honeydew)	

FODMAPs in fruit and vegetables

Food	High in FODMAPs	Moderate levels of FODMAPs	
Vegetables	• asparagus • cauliflower • chicory root • garlic • globe and Jerusalem artichokes • leeks • mangetout • mushrooms (button, chestnut, enoki, porcini, portobello, shiitake) • onions • sauerkraut • seaweed (wakame) • shallots • spring onions (white part) • sprouted chickpeas • sugar snap peas	• 30g (1oz) fresh beetroot • 50g (1¾oz) broccoli stalks • 45g (1¾oz) long-stem broccoli • 3 Brussels sprouts • 60g (2¼oz) butternut squash • celery (less than a third of a stick) • ¾ corn on the cob • 60g (2¼oz) fennel bulb • ¼ green pepper • mangetout (7 pods) • okra (9 pieces) • 18g (c.¾oz) peas • pickled garlic (1 clove) • pickled onions (2 onions, 45g/1¾oz) • 55g (2oz) Savoy cabbage • sugar snap peas (7 pods) • sun-dried tomatoes (4 pieces) • 75g (2¾oz) tinned sweetcorn • 100g (3½oz) sweet potato	

Low in FODMAPs

- alfalfa sprouts
- artichoke hearts
- aubergines
- bamboo shoots
- bean sprouts
- beetroot, pickled
- broccoli florets
- cabbage (white, red)
- carrots
- cassava
- celeriac
- chard
- chicory leaves
- chillies
- Chinese cabbage
- chives
- collard greens
- courgettes
- cucumbers
- edamame beans
- endive leaves
- green beans
- kale
- kohlrabi
- lettuce
- mushrooms (oyster or tinned)
- olives (60g/2¼oz)
- pak choi
- parsnips
- peppers (red, orange, yellow)
- plantain
- potatoes
- pumpkin
- rocket
- seaweed (nori)
- spinach
- spring onions (green part only)
- swede
- Swiss chard
- tomatoes
- turnips
- water chestnuts
- watercress
- yam

FODMAPs in drinks

High-FODMAP	Moderate-FODMAP	Low-FODMAP
• aloe drinks • apple cordial • apple juice • berry smoothies • chai tea, strong • dandelion tea, strong • fennel tea • green tea, strong • herbal tea, strong • malted milk drink • oolong tea, strong • some fruit wines may not be suitable	• <70g (2½oz) buttermilk • 9g (c.¼oz) carob powder • chai tea, weak • <125ml (4fl oz) coconut milk drink • dandelion tea, weak • 120ml (4fl oz) hemp milk drink • herbal tea, weak • <30ml (1fl oz) oat milk drink in UK* • 25ml (scant 1fl oz) orange cordial • 150ml (¼ pint) fresh orange juice • 200ml (7fl oz) rice milk drink • 10ml (2 tsp) rum • 50ml (2fl oz) sweetened soy milk drink • 120ml (4fl oz) unsweetened soy milk from soy beans	• beer • 8g (c.¼oz) cocoa powder • 100ml (3½fl oz) coconut water • cranberry juice • decaffeinated/ caffeinated tea and coffee (see page 111) • gin • 10g (¼oz) hot chocolate powder • 180ml (6¼fl oz) kombucha • peppermint tea • rooibos tea • tomato juice • vegetable juice (tomato and carrot based) • vodka • water, still and sparkling • whisky • wine (red, white and sparkling)

*This may differ between individual countries.

Q: Can I cook for my family with onions/garlic and then remove them from my meal?

Sadly not, as the FODMAPs will leach into the meal. However, you can try using a garlic-infused oil (see pages 132–3) to capture the flavour without the FODMAPs.

Low-FODMAP foods round-up

The table on pages 118–20 shows you all the low-FODMAP foods in one place. This does not include the moderate-FODMAP foods listed elsewhere, but is a useful at-a-glance guide to just how many foods you really can eat during the restriction stage.

Low-FODMAP foods you can eat

Fruit		
• bananas (firm)	• kumquats	• passion fruit
• clementines	• lemons	• pineapples
• 30g (1oz) shredded, dried coconut	• limes	• plantains
	• mandarins	• strawberries
• grapefruit	• <100g (3½oz) melons (cantaloupe and honeydew)	• tangerines
• grapes		• tomatoes
• guava	• oranges	
• jackfruit	• papayas	
• kiwifruit		

Veg		
alfalfa sprouts	courgettes	potatoes
aubergines	cucumbers	pumpkin
bamboo shoots	edamame beans	rocket
bean sprouts	endive leaves	seaweed (nori)
beetroot, pickled	green beans	spinach
broccoli florets	kale	spring onions (green part only)
cabbage (white, red)	kohlrabi	swede
carrots	lettuce	Swiss chard
cassava	mushrooms (oyster or tinned)	turnips
celeriac		water chestnuts
chard	60g (2¼oz) olives	watercress
chicory leaves	pak choi	yam
chillies	parsnips	
Chinese cabbage	peppers (red, orange, yellow)	
chives	plantain	
collard greens		

4. STAGE 1: THE RESTRICTION STAGE

Dairy and dairy substitutes

butter	Gruyère	soy, rice, oat, nut, pea, hemp or quinoa plant drinks (choose fortified versions and check quantities)
Brie	hard cheeses	
Camembert	lactose-free milk	
Cheddar	mozzarella	
coconut yogurt	Parmesan	soy custard
feta	Pecorino	soy yogurt
goats' cheese	Swiss cheese	

Carbohydrates

Bread

bread made using oats, quinoa, maize, millet, buckwheat, cornmeal, rice, potato, tapioca flour

dosa, plain

100% spelt sourdough bread

wheat-free or gluten-free breads (remember to check the label for apple juice or onion/garlic)

wonton wrapper

Flour

rice, potato, gluten-free, buckwheat or tapioca

Rice and pasta

gluten-free couscous

gluten-free gnocchi

gluten-free pasta

polenta

quinoa

quinoa pasta

rice

soba, kelp and rice noodles

100% spelt sourdough pasta

Cereals and grains

buckwheat groats

cornflakes

oats, porridge and oat flakes, oat biscuits

quinoa and rice flakes

rice cereals

Cakes and biscuits

almond and polenta cakes

flourless cakes

gluten-free cakes/biscuits

oat biscuits and flapjacks (check label for flour)

Crackers and snacks

100% buckwheat crackers

corn cakes

gluten-free crackers

oatcakes

rice cakes and crackers

Protein

eggs	<25g (1oz) most nuts and seeds	spirulina
firm tofu (not silken)	2 tbsp nut butter	sprouted mung beans
fish	small amounts of some pulses and beans	tempeh
2 tbsp tinned lentils		
meat	shellfish	
mycoprotein		

Flavourings

capers	mayonnaise	tamarind paste
chilli sauce	mint sauce/jelly	tomato purée
chutney	miso paste	vanilla essence
coconut cream	mustard	vanilla pods
curry powder	nutritional yeast	vinegar
fish sauce	oyster sauce	wasabi powder
most herbs and spices (no onions or garlic)	raspberry jam	Worcestershire sauce
	shrimp paste	
homemade stock	soy sauce	
horseradish sauce	sweet and sour sauce	
ketchup	tahini	

Miscellaneous

agar-agar

arrowroot

baking powder

bicarbonate of soda

cornflour

cream of tartar

Key nutrients of concern

While you may think going on the restriction phase of the low-FODMAP diet will affect your nutritional intake, it is actually perfectly possible to meet all your nutritional needs during this stage. However, the research studies that show us this often involve people being provided with all the food they are going to eat, or being given plenty of dietitian support, so this highlights once again the importance of not attempting to follow this diet on your own.

Fibre

Fibre is a key component in our diets, and gives our gut bacteria food to ferment. Following a low-FODMAP diet is likely to reduce your intake of fibre by up to 4g per day. It is recommended we aim for 30g a day, so this is over a tenth of your total intake. Therefore, it is key to eat high-fibre, low-FODMAP foods. Both high- and low-FODMAP foods can contain a mix of both soluble and insoluble fibre. Here's where fibre gets complicated! Use the table on pages 122–4 for ideas of what you can focus on eating to make sure you are eating enough fibre.

How to eat more fibre on the low-FODMAP diet

Foods	Fibre content	FODMAP content	Ideas
Quinoa	5g per 150g (5½oz) cooked quinoa	low	Try as a carb accompaniment to your meals instead of rice or couscous.
Kiwifruit	5g per 2 kiwifruit (2 = 1 portion)	2 kiwifruit = low	Eat the skin for extra fibre!
Green beans	3.4g in 140g (5oz)	15 beans (140g/5oz) = low	Try roasted with a drizzle of olive oil and a sprinkle of sesame seeds for extra fibre.
Chia seeds	8–10g per 24g (c.1oz/2 tbsp)	low	Add to porridge, sprinkle over yogurt or stir into flapjacks. Chia seeds also contain omega-3 fatty acids, magnesium and calcium.
Chickpeas (tinned, drained and rinsed)	8g per 40g (1½oz)	42g (2 tbsp) = low	Add to casseroles, soups and salads.
Gluten-free multi-seed/ wholegrain bread	1.2g per slice	low	
Oatcakes	4.4g per 4 oatcakes	low	A great snack with nut butter or cheese.

Foods	Fibre content	FODMAP content	Ideas
Oat bisks (Oatibix)	3.4g × 2 bisks	low	Serve with fruit for extra fibre.
Brown rice	3.5g per 135g (4¾oz) cooked	low	Add to soups or salads as well as your usual rice meals.
Flaxseeds	2g per 1 tbsp	1 tbsp = low	Sprinkle over yogurt or add to your breakfast cereal and porridge.
Polenta	6g per 150g (5½oz) cooked	low	Buy this ready cooked and sliced, then grill for a tasty side with a meal.
Lentils, tinned, drained and rinsed	3–5g per 100g (3½oz)	46g (2 tbsp) tinned or 23g (1 tbsp) boiled lentils = medium	Fabulous added to chilli, soups and in place of meat. Also a source of protein and iron.
Kale	2g per 35g (1¼oz)	up to 35g = low	Try this roasted as a snack.
Carrots	2g fibre per 65g (2½oz)	low	Keep them chopped up raw in the fridge for handy snacking.
Oats	4g per 70g (2½oz)	low	So versatile: use for porridge, flapjacks and crumble toppings.

Foods	Fibre content	FODMAP content	Ideas
Oranges	3g per medium orange	low	
Raspberries	4g per 15 raspberries	30 raspberries = low	
Pumpkin Seeds	5g per 30g (1oz)	low	Use in flapjacks, as a topping for yogurt and desserts or add them to porridge.
Pecans	20g per 10 nuts	low	Keep them handy for snacking.
Banana	3g per medium unripe banana	low	
Potato	3g per medium potato	low	Eat the skin for extra fibre!
Broccoli	2.3g per 60g (2¼oz)	low	You can use the stalk too, but keep to a smaller portion as it is higher in FODMAPs.
Bean sprouts	1g per 75g (2¾oz) cup	low	A great addition to stir-fries and salads.
Peanuts	2.4g per 32 nuts	low	

You can eat a medium–high fibre, low-FODMAP diet: it just takes some commitment and planning. Start with oats for breakfast with fruit and seeds, snack on nuts, have quinoa, brown rice, gluten-free wholemeal bread, oatcakes or a skin-on potato with your main meals, along with low-FODMAP vegetables – and don't forget you can add small amounts of some to main meals too. Here's an example of how you can meet a 25–30g daily intake of fibre on a low-FODMAP diet.

Breakfast. 70g (2½oz) oats cooked with milk, topped with pumpkin seeds and raspberries (12g fibre)

Snack: orange (3g fibre)

Lunch: 2 slices of gluten-free multi-seed bread with cheese and tomato, plus carrot sticks, plain crisps and yogurt (5.5g fibre)

Snack: 3 oatcakes with cheese (3.3g fibre)

Evening meal: Salmon and low-FODMAP vegetable stir-fry with brown rice (5g fibre)

Calcium

Calcium intake can be reduced in the short term on the restriction stage of the diet. This is thought to be due to the restriction of lactose and dairy products.[55] As calcium is important for bones, teeth and the nervous system, it is important to ensure you eat calcium-rich foods each day. Plan on eating two to three portions a day (see the table below for information on portions). Check all plant milks and alternatives to yogurt for their calcium content, and remember to give those milk cartons a shake before you pour. Please do not be tempted to make plant milks yourself, as these will not include the added calcium that the commercial products contain. As soon as you can, it is key to reintroduce calcium-rich foods and test your tolerance to them. If you need to restrict lactose, then do make swaps for lactose-free/dairy-free drinks, yogurts and cheeses that have added calcium, at the very least. Most plant-based drinks now have added calcium, vitamin B12 and iodine.

Calcium-rich low-FODMAP foods

Eat two to three portions of calcium-rich foods a day.

Calcium-rich low-FODMAP dairy foods

- 125–150g (4½–5½oz) suitable yogurt
- 200ml (7fl oz) suitable milk (fortified with calcium)
- 30g (1oz) suitable cheese

Calcium-rich low-FODMAP non-dairy foods

- 100–140g (3½–5oz) tinned fish with edible small bones (pilchards, sardines)
- 120g (4¼oz) tofu
- 100–120g (3½–4¼oz) dark green leafy vegetables (spinach, Swiss chard, collard greens, kale)
- sesame seeds (limit to <25g/1oz a day)

- low-FODMAP breakfast cereals fortified with calcium
- 100–140g (3½–5oz) tinned salmon
- 80g (2¾oz) rhubarb

Iron

Iron is another nutrient to be aware of. While it is totally possible to meet your iron needs on the restriction stage of the low-FODMAP diet, it is important to ensure you eat iron-rich foods to replace the iron you might previously have got from fortified breakfast cereals, pulses and nuts.

Tips for iron intake

- Add leafy greens to main meals (spinach, collard greens, chard).
- If you eat meat, include red meat in your diet once or twice a week.
- Tofu is a good source of iron and calcium.
- Use moderate amounts of beans and pulses (see table on page 106).
- Include vitamin C with your meal: it can help aid iron absorption.
- Restrict tea and coffee to between mealtimes, as they can stop you from absorbing as much iron.

Iron-rich low-FODMAP foods

- almonds, hazelnuts, sesame seeds, sunflower seeds*
- broccoli
- butter beans, chickpeas, lentils*

• eggs

• leafy greens (spinach, collard greens, chard)

• peanut butter

• red meat (beef, pork, lamb, liver, sausages)

• tofu

*Please check suitable amounts in the 'FODMAPs in plant-based proteins' table on page 106.

Gluten

This is something that people often cut out as an initial step, thinking it will help with their IBS. However, gluten is not actually a FODMAP. On the low-FODMAP diet, it is wheat rather than gluten itself that is eliminated. It is actually unclear if gluten itself is the direct cause of symptoms, as we rarely just eat gluten on its own. Gluten is the main structural protein in wheat, rye and barley, and it is the protein eliminated in coeliac disease. Some people with IBS may notice a difference to their symptoms when they stop eating gluten. This could be for a number of reasons. It could be that you have undiagnosed coeliac disease. Another possible reason is simply that if you cut out gluten, you will be eating less wheat. In addition, reducing your gluten intake will also reduce your consumption of fructans and FODMAPs, which can therefore improve your symptoms – without the gluten itself being the culprit. Try not to assume gluten is the culprit and stick to the low-FODMAP plan.

Top tips for eating low-FODMAP

Plan your meals

It can feel overwhelming when you start reading all the food lists, so I'd suggest putting those aside for now and just writing out a meal plan for a normal week. If you normally plan your meals anyway, pull out a few weeks' worth. If not, just list all your normal meals, snacks and drinks. Now you can go through these and work out where the FODMAPs are, and what you need to change. Doing this can help things feel more manageable. This can form the basis of your shopping list.

Here are some examples of the kind of changes you might make:

Current food	Change to
Weetabix with 1 banana and cows' milk	Oatibix with 1 firm yellow banana (riper bananas are higher in FODMAPs) and lactose-free milk
Apple and cashew nuts	Orange and 10 almonds
Cheese, pickle and salad sandwich, with crisps, yogurt and a pear	Gluten-free pitta bread with cheese, tomato, cucumber and baby spinach, with plain crisps or popcorn, lactose-free yogurt and a kiwifruit
Tea and biscuits	Tea with lactose-free milk and gluten-free biscuits

Current food	Change to
Spaghetti bolognese with pasta, served with peppers, carrots, broccoli and cheese	Gluten-free spaghetti with bolognese made without onion, garlic or shop-bought stock cubes (instead use the greens of spring onions, asafoetida, homemade stock and mixed dried herbs). Serve with peppers, carrots, broccoli and Cheddar cheese.

Plan out meals for a few weeks, then reuse those meal plans or make up some fresh ones. Use the recipes at the end of this book for inspiration.

Plan your snacks

It can be easy to focus on the main meals but forget the snacks, which could undo all your hard work. Here are some snack ideas:

- Fruit and veggies make great snacks: just remember to stick to the low-FODMAP varieties (see page 118), and keep to one portion of fruit at a time. I always recommend having fruit or veg with either a protein food or a carbohydrate to help stabilize your blood sugars and keep you feeling fuller for longer.

- Oatcakes and gluten-free crackers can make an easier snack than gluten-free bread, as this can have a tendency to fall apart when transported.

- Get baking with some of the recipes in this book: flapjacks, muffins and cookies are all easy to make FODMAP friendly.

- Make smoothies using lactose-free milk and suitable fruit. Add nut butter, seeds or oats for protein or fibre.

Often, snacks and drinks come packed with sweeteners and additives. Here are the ones to look out for:

FODMAPS in sugars

High-FODMAP	Low-FODMAP
agave syrup	aspartame
fructo-oligosaccharides (FOS) and inulin as additives to products	brown sugar
	Canderel
	dark chocolate
fructose, fructose syrup, high-fructose corn syrup	dextrose
fruit juice concentrate	glucose
golden syrup	glucose syrup
honey	icing sugar
malt extract	jaggery
milk and white chocolate	maple syrup
molasses	palm sugar
oligofructose	rice malt syrup
sorghum syrup	saccharin
sugar-free sweets and chocolate (including chewing gum)	Splenda
	stevia
	sucralose
	sucrose
	white sugar

Low-FODMAP snack ideas

- grapes with Cheddar cheese and oatcakes
- suitable berries (up to 20 blueberries or strawberries) and lactose-free yogurt
- plain popcorn sprinkled with cinnamon sugar or herbs and cheese
- oatcakes, gluten-free crackers or rice cakes topped with nut butter, cheese, Marmite, jam, sliced egg or meat
- handful of nuts with 1 tablespoon of raisins
- smoothie made with dairy-free milk, pineapple, raspberries and oats

Cooking tips

While not being able to eat onion, garlic and stock cubes can seem like your meals will become bland, there are so many other great ways to add flavour. Good alternatives for that onion and garlic flavour include asafoetida powder and the green parts of spring onions. Here are a few tips and ideas for adding flavour and variety to your cooking.

Make your own garlic-infused oil

Infuse oil with the flavour of garlic without the FODMAPs. Simply warm some olive, sunflower or vegetable oil in a saucepan over a love heat until warm, not hot. Pop in a couple of peeled cloves of garlic, then remove from the heat and leave for a couple of hours. Now strain the oil through a fine wire mesh strainer or a muslin cloth and remove the garlic cloves. Store the oil for up to three days in the fridge, or freeze it in portions.

Make your own stock

Try making your own stock by boiling up the bones when you have a roast. Add in some vegetable peelings and fresh herbs, and leave it to simmer for a couple of hours. Strain, and you have a homemade stock perfect for adding to your risottos, soups, casseroles and curries. You can keep this in the fridge for three days, or freeze it in portions. It will defrost quickly in the microwave.

To make a vegetable stock, use a mix of low-FODMAP vegetables (such as carrots, fennel leaves and celeriac) plus herbs (such as star anise, parsley stalks, thyme, peppercorns and bay leaf). Simmer in water for 2 hours and strain.

Homemade stock will keep for 3–4 days in the refrigerator and for up to 6 months in the freezer.

Choose the right herbs and spices

Use a variety of herbs and spices to bring your food to life (see the table overleaf). There are so, so many to choose from!

Herbs, spices and flavourings for the low-FODMAP diet

Avoid	OK to use	
Garlic (dried, extract, powder, purée, garlic salt, garlic granules, 'lazy' garlic)	allspice	kaffir lime leaves
	angelica	lemon balm
	anise	lemon and lime juice
	asafoetida	lemongrass
	basil	marjoram
Onion (dried, extract, powder, purée, onion salt)	bay leaf	miso
	black pepper	mustard seeds
	caraway seeds	nigella seed
Check: gravy, stock cubes, soups, sauces, crisps, dressings, ready meals, flavoured breads, pizza	cardamom	nutmeg
	cayenne pepper	nutritional yeast
	chervil	oregano
	chilli	paprika
	chives	parsley
Remember: The phrases 'flavour', 'flavouring' and 'natural flavour' can all mean something contains onion and garlic.	cinnamon	peppermint
	cloves	rosemary
	coriander (leaves and seeds)	saffron
		sage
	cumin	smoked paprika
	curry powder and leaves	soy sauce
	dill	star anise
	fennel seeds	tamarind paste
	fenugreek	tarragon
	fish sauce	thyme
	five spice	turmeric
	galangal	vanilla
	garlic-infused oil (strained so there is no garlic in it)	vinegars (balsamic <1 tbsp)
		wasabi powder
	ginger	Worcestershire sauce
	homemade stock (see page 133)	

Shopping

As someone with personal experience of digestive issues and being wheat-free, I can tell you that the range of foods on offer has vastly improved over the last ten years. Stock up so you are ready for action with:

- herbs and spices (see opposite)
- gluten-free pasta, rice and grains
- gluten-free bread and crackers
- gluten-free pizza bases
- low-FODMAP snacks (gluten-free pretzels, oatcakes, plain popcorn, plain crisps, nuts, seeds)
- low-FODMAP sauces
- tuna, tofu, tempeh and other low-FODMAP protein sources
- gluten-free flour
- eggs
- oats and gluten-free cereal

I know I've said this already, but always check the labels, including those gluten-free products. They can still contain FODMAPs. Planning out your meals will help you with putting together your shopping list. Take your FODMAP booklets or app with you so you can double-check labels in the supermarket.

Eating out

Look at menus online before you go out, and ring up to check the restaurant is happy to accommodate your needs and make swaps.

It may be that they have not heard of the diet before, but are still happy to make changes with your advice, so it's always best to check in advance. Ordering from the gluten-free menu (if one is available) can be easier, but remember that not all gluten-free meals will be suitable, as they may still contain onions and garlic, for example. Also beware of anything cooked with a stock: risotto is often listed on a gluten-free menu, but is made with stock, onions and garlic.

Simple meals without sauces can be a safer and easier choice: see the ideas below. Ask for your meal without sauces and dips, or ask for them to be served on the side, as these are often FODMAP foods.

Suitable low-FODMAP options when eating out

- gluten-free pizza with ham, cheese and peppers (checking for onion or garlic in the tomato sauce)
- rice noodles with meat or tofu/pad Thai (checking for onion, garlic and unsuitable vegetables)
- sushi, sashimi, tempura
- grilled meats or fish with chips/new potatoes and steamed low-FODMAP vegetables
- jacket potato with tuna, mayonnaise on the side and a salad with low-FODMAP vegetables (lettuce, cucumber, pepper, tomatoes)
- gluten-free cheese sandwich with plain crisps and salad
- tandoori dishes with plain rice (no onions or garlic)

If you accidentally end up eating some FODMAPs and have symptoms, do not panic! You have not caused yourself any long-term damage. Just get back to low-FODMAP exclusion and carry on. You don't have to go back to the very beginning: just carry on from where you are. When it comes to the reintroductions, you want to have had at least one week of no symptoms before you start.

What to do if your symptoms have not gone away at the end of the restriction phase

If you have been on the restriction phase of the low-FODMAP diet for eight weeks without seeing any changes, there can be a number of reasons why. Sadly, as I have explained, the low-FODMAP diet is not a magic cure for everyone. While it is very effective for up to 75 per cent of people, there will also always be some people for whom it does not work.

Many people will find that their symptoms reduce but do not fully resolve. It is also good to remember that some level of symptoms of wind and bloating are normal, so do not expect these to totally disappear. It's possible that your symptoms have improved a bit, but if you have not been tracking these closely, it can be easy to forget how bad things were. This is about finding the quality of life that works for you. IBS symptoms also tend to fluctuate and change over time: this can be due

---

to stress, a change in hormone profile, your menstrual cycle, levels of activity or illness.

If you're not seeing any improvement, this is a good point to go back to your dietitian and healthcare team for advice. It could be some FODMAPs have been creeping into your diet and you have been unaware, or that the moderate FODMAPs have stacked up too far. It's also important to talk about other options at this stage. It could be that you do not actually have IBS, but another condition that needs to be explored, or that another therapy is needed, such as CBT or gut-related hypnotherapy.

5. STAGE 2: THE REINTRODUCTION STAGE

Once your symptoms are settled, or at least much improved, it is time to start reintroductions. A key concern for people at this point is that once their symptoms die down, they don't want to risk them starting up again. This fear is understandable, but it can lead to some people staying in the elimination stage for much longer than necessary: even for years. However, as we have discussed, by not reintroducing foods, you risk nutritional inadequacies and gut-health consequences due to the lack of diversity and prebiotic foods, so making these reintroductions is absolutely necessary. While it can cause anxiety to have to reintroduce foods that may lead to your symptoms reappearing, try to keep in mind that this will only be short term. This stage is designed as a series of 'food challenges' through which you reintroduce different foods. You go back on the restriction phase of the low-FODMAP diet between these food challenges, so if you do get any symptoms, this will calm things down again.

This stage takes an average of six to ten weeks if you work through the challenges one at time. This might seem like a long time, but it isn't when you consider the long-term benefits. Remember, it is important that you end up eating as varied a diet as possible to help you meet your body's nutritional needs and to improve your quality of life. The more foods you can add in and the more you can learn about your triggers, the easier things will be. Different people are sensitive to different FODMAPs, so this testing stage is vital to help you discover which foods you can eat to bring you more variety and pleasure in eating.

Q: I've been on the restriction stage of the low-FODMAP diet for a long time without doing the reintroductions. Should I start them now?

Yes, it is important to challenge these foods, but it you have been on the restriction stage of the diet for more than a few months, you may find your body has a heightened reaction to the FODMAPs and you might experience worse symptoms than before when you reintroduce them. So start with half the portion sizes detailed on the following pages and build them up over three to five days until you get to a normal portion size or have moderate–severe symptoms. If you have severe symptoms with a lot of foods, then retry them at a later date.

There are a couple of ways to do the reintroductions. In this book, I'm just going to talk you through the gold standard way. If this is a struggle for you, your dietitian may talk you through the traffic light method or another simple way of doing it.

Understanding the reintroduction stage

Before reintroducing any foods, you need to ensure your symptoms are well controlled. This is why, as you complete the food challenges, you should continue to follow the low-FODMAP diet guidance for all other foods. Each food challenge takes three days to complete, and there are ten main challenges to complete in this stage (see the 'Reintroductions' table on page 148–9). It is important to keep a diary monitoring your symptoms each day, as it is so easy to forget.

Washout days

If you have significant symptoms (symptoms that affect your quality of life) on any of the three-day challenges, that is your sign to stop, note it down and move on to the 'washout' days. This involves returning to the restriction phase of the low-FODMAP diet to remove all FODMAPs from your system and help any symptoms settle down before you try the next challenge food. Even if you do not have any symptoms during a challenge, you still need to remove the challenge food from your diet after three days and complete the washout days before the next challenge. This is so you can be sure which FODMAP group is causing a reaction. You may need more than three washout days if you do have symptoms and they take a while to settle down. Avoid the temptation to rush this stage: it really is worth doing thoroughly.

The reintroduction and personalization stage of the low-FODMAP diet

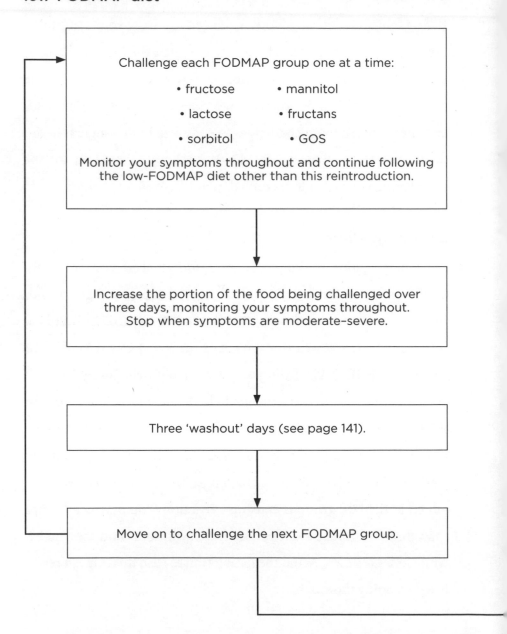

Challenge each FODMAP group one at a time:

- fructose
- mannitol
- lactose
- fructans
- sorbitol
- GOS

Monitor your symptoms throughout and continue following the low-FODMAP diet other than this reintroduction.

Increase the portion of the food being challenged over three days, monitoring your symptoms throughout. Stop when symptoms are moderate–severe.

Three 'washout' days (see page 141).

Move on to challenge the next FODMAP group.

Once all FODMAP groups are tested, bring back each food group according to your tolerance:

• Good tolerance = eat freely

• Medium tolerance = include when you feel able, and don't have too many of these foods at once

• Poorly tolerated = avoid as much as possible

Personalize your diet to ensure you are getting all nutrients.

Keep on reassessing your tolerance and gradually adding in small amounts of fibre and other foods.

How the food challenges work

Day one: small portion/moderate FODMAPs

Eat the food at the correct portion size ('The reintroductions' table on pages 148–9). Make a record of what you eat and write down any symptoms you experience.

If you have significant symptoms, stop at this point and go back to the low-FODMAP diet for two to three days or until your symptoms have cleared.

If there were no significant symptoms, you are fine with a small amount of that FODMAP and can move on to the next stage.

Day two: medium portion/high FODMAPs

Now move on to the next portion size. Again, write it down and record any symptoms.

If you have significant symptoms, stop at this point and go back to the low-FODMAP diet for two to three days or until your symptoms have cleared.

If you are symptom-free, proceed to the next stage.

Day three: large portion/very high FODMAPs

Move on to the next portion size and record any symptoms.

You do not need to have as large a portion size if it feels like more than you could normally manage, but doing it this way does give an absolute test.

Days four to seven: washout period

Go back to the low-FODMAP diet for two to three days or until your symptoms settle. Then you can move on to the next challenge. Remember: you need still have to complete the washout days even if you didn't have symptoms. The FODMAPs can still build up in your system, and we want to start with a FODMAP-free gut when testing each food.

Monitoring your symptoms

I cannot stress enough how important it is to write down what you eat, the amount and any IBS symptoms you experience. It can also be helpful to note if there was anything else different happening that day, for example an extra-stressful day at work, a yoga session, or a meal out. If you have symptoms after eating a food, it is essential to record the amount you ate. You are going to want to look back at this at the end. As a dietitian, I can assure you that food diaries are worth their weight in gold!

Example of a food and symptoms diary

Date	FODMAP tested	Amount eaten	Symptoms	Stress levels
10/5/21	Mango	¼ mango	None	Normal
11/5/21	Mango	½ mango	Some bloating and looser stools, opened bowels twice	Normal
12/5/21	Mango	1 mango	More bloating, tummy felt upset and I had to go to the bathroom 4 times with loose stools	Normal

This diary shows us that the person can definitely tolerate one quarter of a mango, and could possibly tolerate half a mango on some days, depending on what else they have eaten.

Testing the individual FODMAP groups

The table overleaf gives a suggested order in which you can work through the FODMAP challenges, you can do this in a different order if you wish. Just choose which FODMAP group you want to start with. Think about the foods you have missed the most. Often, people tell me that they've missed wheat, onions and garlic. If that's the case for you too, start with the fructans group. Work through the groups in the order that suits you best.

A few notes before you begin:

- Foods containing GOS, lactose and fructose can all be tested using just one food challenge to cover the whole group. Test them using a food that is high in that FODMAP group. If you react, you are likely to have a problem with all foods in that group. If you are able to tolerate a certain amount, then note this down ready for stage 3.
- Polyols need to be tested in two subgroups: sorbitol and mannitol.
- You only need to test the foods that you normally eat. If there are foods you never eat, there is no point in testing them.
- The gut handles different fructan-containing foods differently, which means you will need to challenge each fructan food separately. Begin by testing wheat and onion/garlic, then move on to the other fructans (see 'Testing the remaining fructans' on pages 150–1). This is a bit of a pain, but it will give you a clearer answer as to what is causing your symptoms.
- With all foods you test, monitor for any symptoms and write them down in whatever way works for you! Use a notebook, a spreadsheet or one of the apps listed in the Resources (see pages 247–8).

The reintroductions

Challenge number*	FODMAP being tested	Recommended foods to use
1	Fructose	Honey or mango
2	Lactose	Cows' milk or natural yogurt
3	Sorbitol	Avocado or corn on the cob
4	Mannitol	Celery or sweet potato
5	Fructans (grains)	Bread (made with wheat)
6	Fructans (grains)	Pasta
7	Fructans (grains)	Breakfast cereal (containing wheat)
8	Fructans (onion)	Onion (test raw onion on day 1: if this is not well tolerated, try cooked onion)
9	Fructans (garlic)	Garlic
10	GOS	Choose one of these: almonds chickpeas peas

*This can be done in a different order.

5. STAGE 2: THE REINTRODUCTION STAGE

Day 1	Day 2	Day 3 (can be split over all your meals)
1½ tsp	2 tsp	1 tbsp
¼ fruit	½ fruit	1 fruit
60ml (4 tbsp)	125ml (4fl oz)	250ml (9fl oz)
85g (3oz)	170g (5¾oz)	200g (7oz)
¼ fruit	½ fruit	¾ fruit
½ cob	1 cob	1½ cobs
½ stick	1 stick	1½ sticks
105g (c.3½oz)	140g (5oz)	210g (7½oz)
1 slice	1½ slices	2 slices
99g (c.3½oz)	148g (c.5½oz)	222g (c.8oz)
2 tbsp/1 bisk	4 tbsp/2 bisks	6 tbsp/3 bisks
⅛ onion	¼ onion	½ onion
¼ clove	½ clove	1 clove
15 nuts	20 nuts	30 nuts
45g (1¾oz)	90g (3¼oz)	180g (6¼oz)
18g (c.¾oz)	36g (c.1¼oz)	72g (c.2½oz)

Q: *I don't like the foods in the challenges: can I swap them?*

In the table on pages 148–9, I have given the standard foods used for the reintroduction challenges. There are some alternative foods that can be used for each FODMAP – for example, with fructans, you could use fresh figs, sugar snap peas or sun-dried tomatoes. This is not always standard procedure, though, so do check with your dietitian first to make sure you choose the right food and test with the correct amounts.

Testing the remaining fructans

Now you have worked through each individual group, it's time to challenge the fructan foods individually – but remember, you only need to challenge the ones you eat. Don't forget that these quantities can be spread out over the day if you don't want to eat them all in one go. Here are some examples but you can individualize this to your normal portions.

5. STAGE 2: THE REINTRODUCTION STAGE

Fructan	Day 1	Day 2	Day 3
Fruits			
Currants	1 tbsp	2 tbsp	3 tbsp
Dates	1 date	2 dates	3 dates
Dried figs	1 fig	2 figs	3 figs
Grapefruit	½ medium	1 medium	1 large
Pomegranate	½ small pomegranate	1 small pomegranate	2 small pomegranates
Raisins	1 tbsp	2 tbsp	3 tbsp
Goji berries	1 tbsp	2 tbsp	3 tbsp
Dried cranberries	1 tbsp	2 tbsp	3 tbsp
Vegetables			
Beetroot, fresh	3 slices	4 slices	6 slices
Brussels sprouts	3	4	5
Okra	5	10	15
Savoy cabbage	50g (1¾oz)	70g (2½oz)	100g (3½oz)

Q: I had no symptoms.
Should I test with an even bigger portion?

You can do that if you wish, but think about the amount of the food you would eat in real life. If you are going to end up testing with an amount you would never actually eat, there is no real point.

Q: Help nothing seems to have worked –
I can't eat any foods!

Think about whether you have been strictly following the diet, or whether there have been a lot of slip-up days? If you have been strict, remember that the low-FODMAP diet doesn't work for everyone. It might be time to go back to your GP and ask for some psychological support, or try yoga or gut-related hypnotherapy. It is also a good idea to chat to your dietitian to see if there is another approach they want to try to test for extra food sensitivities.

Top tips for reintroductions

- Choose days where life is calmer and you have a more stable eating pattern. It is best not to test your reintroductions while eating out.
- Plan how you will eat the foods. Will you integrate them into your meals, or will you eat them as extras on the side?
- Always stick to the low-FODMAP diet (other than the particular food challenge you are completing). You are only reintroducing one food at a time, then removing it again.

- You should only put all safe foods back in your diet once you have completed all the food challenges.
- Each food challenge should be done over three consecutive days so that you build up the amount of that FODMAP in your system.
- You should be aiming to build up to an amount of food that reflects your normal portion size, or slightly larger. Remember: any FODMAP consumed in very large amounts is likely to lead to symptoms.
- As soon as you get moderate–severe symptoms, you should stop the challenge you're on and move on to 'washout' days (see page 141).
- You do not need to eat the challenge food all in one meal: it can be spread out over your day.
- Keep your daily caffeine and alcohol intake to sensible limits that do not trigger your IBS.
- If you feel anxious about this stage, then please do chat to your dietitian as there are adjustments that can be made to help you, such as using smaller amounts of the foods or doing the challenges over a longer period of time.
- If you are unsure about your symptoms – maybe you had a stressful day or just forgot to note it down – you can test the same amount for another day to check.

6. STAGE 3: THE PERSONALIZATION STAGE

The personalization stage of the low-FODMAP diet is the exciting part! Now you get to work out your own personal FODMAP plan. This will help you to know exactly what you can and cannot eat in order to help manage your IBS symptoms. While all FODMAPs are potential triggers, the effect different ones have on you will vary, and will also change depending on how much of a particular FODMAP you eat, how often you eat it, and whether you eat it with other FODMAPs. It could be that you can include certain FODMAPs daily in your diet, while you need to eat others less often.

Further testing

You can use the 'FODMAP groups' table overleaf to help you decide whether you want to test more foods in an individual FODMAP group. For example, if you were really sensitive to the bean you tested for the GOS challenge, but tend to eat beans and pulses a lot, you may want to test different types of beans to see if there are some you have a better tolerance level for.

The FODMAP groups

Lactose	custard; ice cream (remember to check ingredients for other FODMAPs); low-fat soft cheese; milk (cows', sheep's, goats'); yogurt (remember to check additional ingredients)
GOS	borlotti beans; butter beans; chickpeas; lentils
Fructose	agave; broad beans; fresh fig; fruit juice (more than 100ml/3½fl oz); honey; larger portions of fruit; mango
Sorbitol	avocados; blackberries; coconuts; corn on the cob; lychees
Mannitol	cauliflower; celery; enoki mushrooms; portobello mushrooms; shiitake mushrooms; sweet potatoes

Mixing FODMAPs

Some foods and meals contain a mix of FODMAPs, and when eaten together, they have a cumulative, stacking effect. If there are foods in the table overleaf that you eat a lot of regularly, it is worthwhile challenging those foods individually. However, challenging every single food will take a very long time, and you will probably end up giving up. The key is to strike a balance between testing enough foods so you know what you can eat and what to avoid, without making the testing stage super longwinded. With the foods you do not test, it can be helpful to just know which FODMAPs they contain, so you can bear this in mind as you experiment with mixed foods and meals in order to work out your individual tolerance. If you know you are more sensitive to GOS, then you may need to be more careful with butternut squash, cashews, pistachios, mangetout and peas, for example.

If you do decide to challenge any of the foods containing multiple FODMAPs that are listed overleaf, use the testing process outlined in the last chapter (including washout days), and increase the quantities as follows:

Day 1: small portion

Day 2: medium portion

Day 3: large portion

Foods containing multiple FODMAPs

FODMAPS	Foods
fructose and sorbitol	apples cherries pears and dried pears tinned apricots
fructans and sorbitol	dried apricots nectarines peaches plums
fructans and fructose	asparagus tinned guava Jerusalem artichoke sultanas
fructans, mannitol and fructose	watermelon
fructans and GOS	amaranth barley cashews peas pistachios
fructans, sorbitol and fructose	coconut flour
mannitol and GOS	butternut squash
fructans, mannitol and GOS	mangetout
fructans and mannitol	button mushrooms

Personalizing your plan

Finding your threshold

Now you can start eating all the foods that you tested that did not give you symptoms. This can take some adjustment, as up until now, you have only tested one food at a time. As you introduce two foods that individually gave you no symptoms or mild symptoms, it could lead to you experiencing moderate symptoms as their FODMAPs stack up. It is advisable to take this stage slowly, as including more than one FODMAP food in a meal will increase the chances of your symptoms being triggered. You will, therefore, need to find your own FODMAP threshold: this is the level of FODMAPs you can include in a meal, day or week without triggering symptoms. Everyone is different, and so your FODMAP threshold is unique. The only way to work it out is to start eating foods and carefully monitor your body's response.

Now you can also start to increase the amounts of moderate-FODMAP foods you eat. Carefully increase your portions of these and record any symptoms. The Monash University FODMAP Diet app (see Resources, page 247) has filters that can help you see which foods you can include in your diet, including the specific amounts you can have. This is very much a trial-and-error approach, which I know can be frustrating – but you are so almost there!

As with stage 2, you may feel some anxiety as you reintroduce foods, but generally most people will not have symptoms to the degree they were having them before starting the low-FODMAP diet

– and now you know that you can reduce those symptoms by going back to the restriction stage of the diet. If you do need to go back on to stage 1 at any point, you can do this as a 'washout' period for a few days, just to relieve any symptoms. Remember, as you start to expand your range and eat mixed meals, you may notice more symptoms. Try building up these foods to work out how much of them you can tolerate. It may be that you can eat chickpeas once a week, but not daily, or that you can have apples and onions on the same day, but adding another FODMAP would send you over your tolerance level.

You may find that you are OK when you first start reintroducing FODMAPs, but that after a few weeks your symptoms return, even though you haven't changed your diet. This can be due to those FODMAPs building up in your system over time. If this happens, you will need to take a washout period and then reintroduce FODMAPs at a lower level – or you may find the best option for you is to just have some FODMAP-free days each week. Some people are able to eat FODMAPs daily; for others it can be just a couple of meals a week.

This whole process takes time and effort, but it is so worthwhile, as it will help you to build the diversity in your diet you need in order to meet your nutritional needs and look after your gut health.

Tracking your progress

As with stage 2, keeping a food and symptoms diary throughout this process is very useful to help you reflect on the links between any symptoms you experience and the foods you've tried, as well as any potential stacking of FODMAPs.

Increasing fibre

As we saw earlier, it can be tricky to get enough fibre on a low-FODMAP diet. At this stage, you can start working on gradually increasing your intake of fibre-containing foods. Do this in small quantities over time so your digestive system adapts. Again, this is something your dietitian can advise on, by sitting down with you and working out a plan of which foods to work on. Aim to eat a wide variety of fruit, vegetables and wholegrains throughout your week. You may be able to slowly increase your intake of fibre and prebiotic foods to work towards the target of 30g fibre a day.

Re-challenging foods

Once you feel you have found your new modified FODMAP diet, you may want to re-challenge certain foods. These could be foods that you have previously tested and had a mild reaction to, or foods you had a stronger reaction to, but really want to be able to eat. This is all part of the personalization stage, which can take time, but will hopefully leave you with more variety in your diet.

You can try re-challenging the foods by using smaller portions, as you may find that you can manage a smaller dose than the one used in the initial food challenges. For example, if there is a food you love, but you had symptoms on day one of the challenge, try retesting it with half the day one amount, then three-quarters of it, then the full day-one portion.

It may be helpful to revisit the challenge foods at a later date, as our tolerances to food can change over time, and you may find your reaction to the food is now different.

You can also try different forms of the same food. If whole chickpeas give you symptoms, for example, you may find that you are OK with mashed-up or processed chickpeas in the form of hummus.

Think about testing other trigger foods that you may have cut out, including caffeine, fatty foods, alcohol and spices. It may be that you have tested these previously as part of the first-line advice so already know the answers to this. If you haven't, try testing these foods now. Begin with a small amount on day one, double it for day two, and triple it for day three. Remember, you can spread this amount out over the whole day. As with some of the FODMAPs, you may find you can tolerate some of these 'trigger' foods in smaller quantities.

You will end up with a diet that is personalized for you. How amazing is that?

Finding a balance

Remember that everyone's FODMAP tolerance is different and the FODMAPs will all add up. If you eat too many in a short period of time, you may experience symptoms. But you can also use this information to your advantage. If there are specific foods that you know give you symptoms, but you still want to eat occasionally, try having them on days you do not eat many other FODMAPs and keep the portions small. Or simply be aware that you can choose to eat these foods and know that you may have symptoms afterwards. Sometimes it can be worth it just to enjoy a food you've missed, and it is not going to cause your gut any damage.

While eating fewer FODMAPs can help you feel better, it is important not get obsessive about it. Stress and anxiety can have a huge impact on your IBS symptoms, so striking a balance between eating your own personalized FODMAP diet and also being able to enjoy life is important. If you do eat something that you know may cause you symptoms, instead of feeling anxious about it, why not treat it as a chance to re-test that food? It could be that you are now able to eat it.

It is also key to remember that your tolerances to food can change and your IBS symptoms may flare up from time to time. This can be caused by a number of things, including stress and anxiety (as mentioned above), pregnancy, or just being at a different stage in life. If this happens, you can go back to stage 1 of the low-FODMAP diet for a couple of weeks, and you can also revisit the first-line advice, but then do make sure you return to your personalized diet and reintroduce all the foods that you were eating. Remember, it is important for your gut health and overall nutritional intake to eat as varied a diet as possible.

Gut health

Before we finish, it's time to revisit your gut health, as this is an important part of your long-term plan. The low-FODMAP diet is known to affect the gut microbiota. A study on 27 IBS subjects and 6 healthy controls showed that 21 days on an extra-low-FODMAP diet reduced the total amount of bacteria in faeces by 47 per cent, and the prebiotic bacteria present in the gut was lower too. The level of butyrate-producing bacteria was also reduced. This shows that eating a higher FODMAP diet can result in a better balance of bacteria in the gut.[56] Other research studies confirm that reducing the FODMAP content of your diet alters the types and amounts of microbes in your gut and faeces. A UK study showed that following a low-FODMAP diet for four weeks improved symptoms, but also reduced the amount of beneficial *bifidobacteria* in the gut, measured through stool samples.[57] With all the research put together, we can be pretty certain that following a low-FODMAP diet will modify your microbiome, and that being on a low-FODMAP diet long term is therefore not a good plan for your overall health.

FODMAPs are fermentable substrates: food for your gut bacteria, if you like. Some FODMAPs (certain fructans and galacto-oligosaccharides) are prebiotics. These are indigestible carbohydrate foods that are fermented in the gut and feed the gut bacteria. This helps stimulate the growth and/or activity of certain microbes in the gut bacteria.[58] At low doses, these prebiotics can encourage the growth of beneficial bacteria in the gut, but this needs to be balanced against the impact of the FODMAPs on your IBS symptoms. This is where working with a highly trained dietitian is beneficial, and also why the reintroductions of these foods, to your tolerance, is so important. You may need to slowly increase these prebiotic foods over time in during stage 3 of this diet. While you are in the restriction stage, you still want to include some low-FODMAP prebiotic foods, and you may find that taking a probiotic helps lessen the effects (see below). A probiotic can help bring up those beneficial bacteria levels.[59]

Low-FODMAP prebiotic foods

Fruit/vegetable	Carbohydrates	Proteins
banana (less than ½, unripe) currants (1 tbsp) pomegranate (½ small fruit) raisins (1 tbsp)	amaranth buckwheat corn couscous multigrain gluten-free bread oats spelt pasta	chickpeas (2 tbsp) boiled red and green lentils (1 tbsp) tinned lentils (2 tbsp) other beans and pulses (to tolerance)
beetroot (2 slices) butternut squash (less than 3 tbsp) cassava (less than 4 tbsp) potatoes pumpkin Savoy cabbage sweetcorn (1 tbsp)		almonds (fewer than 10) hazelnuts (fewer than 10)

Note: Portions have been given for moderate-FODMAP foods. Normal portions can be eaten of all other foods.

It could be that in the future, we will be able to test your microbiome, know which species of bacteria you are low in, and simply give you a top-up with probiotics, or know which specific FODMAPs you need to restrict to help your symptoms. We still have a lot to learn in this exciting area. One big question is how reintroducing FODMAPs helps, and if doing the low-FODMAP diet with a probiotic or prebiotic supplement helps. As always with science, there are so many questions and it is constantly evolving.

Should I take a probiotic while on the low-FODMAP diet?

There are so many probiotics on the market right now, all with different amounts and types of bacteria in them, which makes this a tricky area to navigate. How do you know what bacteria your gut needs? The simple answer is that we can't be certain, but we can be led by the research studies. Right now, the evidence we have suggests that probiotics are unlikely to provide substantial benefit to IBS symptoms, but this doesn't mean they won't help you in other ways. As we have seen, research studies show levels of *Bifidobacteria* and other beneficial gut bacteria are lower in people on the low-FODMAP diet.[60] This could be because many FODMAPs are prebiotic foods that can feed the gut bacteria. Adding a probiotic while on the low-FODMAP diet can help increase *Bifidobacteria* back to nearly normal levels. So it could be that taking a probiotic alongside following the low-FODMAP diet is helpful in the longer term. If you do want to try a probiotic, you should trial one for four weeks and stop if you do not find it beneficial. Always work with your healthcare professional on this, as you want to make sure you are taking a probiotic containing the right strain of bacteria. Some probiotics can actually contain FODMAPs and other ingredients that make them unsuitable for the restriction phase of the diet. Check the label for FOS, inulin, GOS, fructose, sorbitol, xylitol, lactose and fibre.

What should I do about prebiotics on the diet?

The restriction phase of the low-FODMAP diet reduces the levels of prebiotic foods you eat and also reduces fermentable fibre, both of which feed the gut bacteria. While this can help reduce your symptoms in the short term, it provides less food for the gut bacteria, and could be the cause of reduced levels of beneficial *Bifidobacteria* in the gut, which is not a good long-term plan for your health.[61] The key here is to find the right prebiotic foods, as some studies show us that eating prebiotic foods on their own can help IBS symptoms.[62] Ideally, we want a prebiotic that increases the levels of *Bifidobacteria* and leads to more butyrate production, but doesn't trigger IBS symptoms. Inulin is a prebiotic and also a FODMAP: in doses of more than 6g a day, it will increase flatulence and not help IBS symptoms, so stay away from that one. Beta galacto-oligosaccharide, pectin and partially hydrolyzed guar gum, however, may help.[63] The best way to increase prebiotics in your diet is to reintroduce those FODMAPs that are also prebiotics, but remember that not all FODMAPs will work for everyone. Increasing the diversity of your diet is a lot simpler than reading all the research trials on which prebiotic to take!

7. THE RECIPES

While most of the ingredients used in the following recipes are low in FODMAPs, some moderate-FODMAP ingredients feature too. These have been used in safe quantities and highlighted with an asterisk for your convenience.

BREAKFAST

Bacon & maple syrup pancakes

Serves 4

300g (10½oz) gluten-free plain flour

2½ teaspoons gluten-free baking powder

½ teaspoon salt

1 egg, lightly beaten

425ml (15fl oz) lactose-free or plant-based milk (such as coconut, hemp, quinoa, rice, almond or hazelnut)

25g (1oz) butter or margarine, melted

olive oil spray, for oiling

8 smoked back bacon rashers
a drizzle of maple syrup, to serve

Preheat the oven to 150°C/300°F/Gas Mark 2.

Sift the flour, baking powder and salt into a bowl. Mix together, then make a well in the centre and gradually beat in the egg and milk. Continue to beat until the mixture forms a smooth batter. Stir in the melted butter or margarine.

Heat a heavy-based frying pan over a medium heat until hot. Spray lightly with olive oil and spoon in about 100ml (3½fl oz) of the pancake batter. Cook for 1–2 minutes until bubbles start appearing on the surface. Carefully flip the pancake over and cook for a further 1–2 minutes on the other side until browned. Remove from the pan and place on a heatproof plate in the oven to keep warm while you cook the remainder of the batter – it should make 8 pancakes in total.

Meanwhile, preheat the grill to high and cook the bacon for 2 minutes on each side until crispy.

Serve topped with the bacon and drizzled with maple syrup.

Berry & coconut quinoa

Serves 4

175g (6oz) quinoa
300ml (½ pint) lactose-free or plant-based milk (such as coconut, hemp, quinoa, rice, almond or hazelnut)
100ml (3½fl oz) water
100g (3½oz) raspberries
¼ teaspoon ground cinnamon

To serve:
100g (3½oz) blueberries*
a sprinkling of desiccated coconut*
a drizzle of maple syrup

Place the quinoa in a saucepan over a medium heat with the milk, water, raspberries and cinnamon. Bring to the boil, then reduce the heat to low and simmer for 12–15 minutes until the liquid is absorbed and the quinoa is cooked. Serve topped with the blueberries and desiccated coconut and drizzled with maple syrup.

Berry & yogurt pots

Makes 4
400g (14oz) mixed low-FODMAP frozen berries (such as raspberries and strawberries), defrosted
juice of 1 orange
6 tablespoons maple syrup
400ml (14fl oz) lactose-free or plant-based low-FODMAP natural yogurt
50g (1¾oz) Homemade granola (see pages 177–8)

Place half the berries in a blender with the orange juice and maple syrup and whizz until fairly smooth.

Transfer to a bowl and stir in the remaining berries.

Divide a third of the berry mixture between 4 small bowls. Top with half the yogurt, followed by another third of the berry mixture, then the remaining yogurt.

Top with the remaining berry mixture and sprinkle over the granola just before serving.

Bircher muesli

Serves 4

200g (7oz) porridge oats

100g (3½oz) mixed low-FODMAP nuts (such as peanuts, walnuts and macadamia nuts), toasted and roughly chopped

1 tablespoon maple syrup, plus extra to serve

600ml (20fl oz) lactose-free or plant-based milk (such as coconut, hemp, quinoa, rice, almond or hazelnut)

To serve:

150g (5½oz) mixed low-FODMAP berries (such as raspberries and strawberries)

lactose-free or plant-based low-FODMAP natural yogurt

Put the oats and nuts in a bowl and stir in the maple syrup.

Add the milk to the oat-and-nut mixture. Leave to soak for at least 2 hours (or even overnight in the refrigerator).

Serve topped with the mixed berries, yogurt and maple syrup.

Raspberry & mint smoothie

Serves 1 (makes 250ml/9fl oz)

100g (3½oz) frozen raspberries

150ml (¼ pint) lactose-free or plant-based milk (such as coconut, hemp, quinoa, rice, almond or hazelnut)

small bunch of mint

Put the raspberries in a food processor or blender and pour in the milk. Pull the mint leaves off their stalks, reserving a sprig for decoration, and add the leaves to the blender. Whizz until smooth.

Pour the smoothie into a glass, decorate with the reserved mint sprig and serve immediately.

Blueberry & oat bars

Makes 12

100g (3½oz) gluten-free plain wholemeal flour
75g (2¾oz) gluten-free self-raising flour
175g (6oz) butter or margarine, plus extra for greasing
½ teaspoon ground cinnamon
175g (6oz) porridge oats
150g (5½oz) light muscovado sugar
200g (7oz) blueberries*
vanilla sugar, for sprinkling

Preheat the oven to 180°C/350°F/Gas Mark 4 and grease a 28 × 18cm (11 × 7 inch) shallow baking tin.

Put the flours in a bowl or food processor. Add the butter or margarine and rub in with your fingertips or process until the mixture resembles breadcrumbs. Add the cinnamon, oats and muscovado sugar and stir or blend briefly until the mixture forms coarse crumbs and starts to cling together.

Tip about half the mixture into the prepared tin in an even layer. Pack down with the back of a spoon to make a firm base. Scatter over the blueberries and sprinkle over the remaining crumble mixture.

Bake for about 50 minutes–1 hour until the crumble is deep golden. Leave to cool in the tin, then sprinkle with vanilla sugar and cut into bars. The bars will keep in an airtight container for up to 4 days.

Boiled egg with mustard soldiers

Serves 4

2 teaspoons wholegrain mustard, or to taste
50g (1¾oz) unsalted butter, softened
4 large eggs
4 thick slices of multigrain gluten-free low-FODMAP bread
black pepper
mustard and cress, to serve

In a small bowl, beat together the wholegrain mustard and butter. Season with black pepper.

Cook the eggs in a saucepan of boiling water over a medium heat for 4–5 minutes until softly set. Meanwhile, toast the bread, then butter one side with the mustard butter and cut into fingers.

Serve the eggs with the soldiers and some mustard and cress.

Cinnamon & maple syrup porridge

Serves 4

200g (7oz) rolled oats
½ teaspoon ground cinnamon
750ml (1⅓ pints) water or lactose-free or plant-based milk
   (such as coconut, hemp, quinoa, rice, almond or hazelnut)

To serve:

100g (3½oz) raspberries
a drizzle of maple syrup

In a small saucepan, mix together the rolled oats, cinnamon and water or milk.

Cook over a medium heat for 8–9 minutes, stirring occasionally, until thickened. Serve topped with the raspberries and maple syrup.

Eggs Benedict with hollandaise

Serves 2
2 large eggs
1 gluten-free English muffin, halved horizontally and toasted
a little butter or margarine
4 slices of Parma ham
salt and black pepper

For the hollandaise sauce:
1 large egg yolk
1 teaspoon lemon juice
1 teaspoon white wine vinegar
50g (1¾oz) butter or margarine

To make the hollandaise sauce, put the egg yolk in a small food processor or blender and season well with salt and pepper. Heat the lemon juice and vinegar in a small saucepan over a medium heat until just boiling. Switch on the food processor or blender and gradually add the hot vinegar mixture in a steady stream. Turn off the food processor or blender. In the same pan, quickly melt the butter, then turn on the food processor or blender and add the melted butter in a steady stream, as before, to give a smooth sauce.

Bring a large frying pan full of water to the boil, then reduce the heat to a bare simmer. Break the eggs into the water and allow to cook very gently for 2 minutes. Remove from the pan with a slotted spoon.

Butter the muffin halves and top each one with 2 slices of ham, a poached egg and a generous dollop of the hollandaise sauce.

Fruit-stuffed pancakes

Serves 4

115g (4oz) rice flour

1 teaspoon gluten-free baking powder

½ teaspoon ground cinnamon

1 egg

finely grated zest of 1 lemon

175ml (6fl oz) lactose-free or plant-based milk (such as coconut, hemp, quinoa, rice, almond or hazelnut)

2–3 teaspoons sunflower oil

100g (3½oz) strawberries, hulled and halved

100g (3½oz) raspberries

¼ cantaloupe melon, deseeded and chopped

5–6 mint leaves, shredded

4 tablespoons maple syrup

lactose-free or plant-based low-FODMAP yogurt, to serve

Place the flour, baking powder, cinnamon, egg, lemon zest and milk in a food processor. Add 2–3 tablespoons of water, then blend to make a smooth batter.

Heat half the oil in a frying pan over a medium heat. Pour in a quarter of the pancake batter and cook for 2–3 minutes, then flip the pancake over and cook for a further 1–2 minutes on the other side. Remove from the pan and set aside on a warm plate. Repeat with the remaining batter to make three more pancakes, adding more oil to the pan if needed.

In a bowl, gently mix together the fruit. Divide the fruit mixture between the pancakes, placing it in the middle of each one, and sprinkle over some shredded mint. Fold the pancakes in half and place on a baking sheet. Drizzle over the maple syrup.

Preheat the grill to high and grill the folded pancakes for 2–3 minutes. Serve with a dollop of yogurt.

Homemade granola

Serves 4

30g (1oz) maple syrup
1 tablespoon sunflower oil
1 tablespoon warm water
45g (1¾oz) dark muscovado sugar
110g (3¾oz) jumbo oats
55g (2oz) walnut halves
30g (1oz) macadamia nuts, chopped
25g (1oz) dried cranberries*
25g (1oz) desiccated coconut*

To serve:

lactose-free or plant-based low-FODMAP yogurt
mixed low-FODMAP berries (such as raspberries and
  strawberries)

Preheat the oven to 150°C/300°F/Gas Mark 3.

In a bowl, whisk together the maple syrup, oil, warm water and sugar. Stir in the remaining ingredients, except the dried cranberries and coconut, and mix well. Place the mixture on a baking sheet and spread it out evenly. Bake for 15 minutes, then add the dried cranberries and coconut and bake for a further 10 minutes. Remove from the oven and transfer to another baking sheet to cool. Leave to cool completely, then store in an airtight container for up to 1 month.

Serve with yogurt and fresh berries.

Cranberry, orange & carrot juice

Serves 2 (makes about 350ml/12fl oz)
1 orange (about 200g/7oz), roughly peeled
225g (8oz) fresh cranberries*
2 carrots (about 300g/10½oz in total), peeled

Place all the ingredients in a juicer and juice until smooth.

Pour the juice into glasses and serve immediately.

Kedgeree with soft-poached eggs

Serves 4
50g (1¾oz) butter or margarine
6 spring onions (green parts only), chopped
2 tablespoons mild curry powder
300g (10½oz) basmati rice
300ml (½ pint) homemade chicken stock (see page 133)
250g (9oz) smoked haddock, skinned and cut into chunks
200ml (7fl oz) whipping cream
3 tablespoons chopped flat-leaf parsley
1 tablespoon white wine vinegar or malt vinegar
4 very fresh large eggs
1 lemon, cut into wedges
salt and pepper

Melt the butter in a large saucepan over a medium heat. Add the spring onions and fry until soft. Add the curry powder and fry for a further minute until fragrant, then add the rice to the pan and stir well.

Pour in the stock and bring to the boil, then reduce the heat and simmer for 7–10 minutes, or until the rice is just cooked. Add the smoked haddock, cream and parsley. Cook for a further 2 minutes until the fish is cooked and firm. Season with salt and pepper.

Bring a large saucepan of water to the boil. Add the vinegar and a pinch of salt. Whisk the water around the pan, then crack the first egg into the centre of the spiral of water. Reduce the heat to low and simmer for 2–3 minutes until the white of the egg is set but the yolk is still soft. Remove from the pan using a slotted spoon and plunge the egg into a bowl of ice-cold water to stop it from cooking further. Repeat with the remaining eggs. Once all the eggs are cooked, bring the water in the pan back up to a simmer and return the eggs to the pan for 1 minute to warm through.

Serve the hot kedgeree topped with the poached eggs, with lemon wedges on the side for squeezing.

Ranch eggs

Serves 4

1 tablespoon garlic-infused olive oil (see pages 132–3)
1 bunch of spring onions (green parts only), sliced
1–2 red chillies, deseeded, if liked, and chopped
2 × 400g (14oz) cans chopped tomatoes
pinch of brown sugar

3 plum tomatoes, thickly sliced

4 eggs

75g (2¾oz) Lancashire cheese, crumbled

chopped coriander leaves

4 soft wheat-free, low-FODMAP corn tortillas

salt and pepper

Preheat the oven to 230°C/450°F/Gas Mark 8.

Heat the garlic-infused oil in a large frying pan over a medium heat. Add the spring onions and cook for 5 minutes until softened. Stir in the chillies and cook for a further 1 minute. Add the tinned tomatoes and sugar and bring to the boil, then season. Reduce the heat to low and simmer for 10 minutes, topping up with water if necessary.

Add the plum tomatoes and cook for 3 minutes. Using the sliced tomatoes as a base, form 4 indentations in the sauce. Crack an egg into each one, then cover the pan with a lid or piece of foil. Increase the heat to medium and cook for about 5 minutes, or until the egg whites are opaque and cooked through.

Remove the lid or foil and scatter over the crumbled cheese and chopped coriander. Place the tortillas on a baking sheet in the oven for 3–5 minutes to warm and soften.

To serve, spoon some of the tomato-and-egg mixture into each tortilla and enjoy straight away.

High-fibre gluten-free buckwheat bread

Makes 1 loaf
450g (1lb) buckwheat flour, plus extra for dusting

3 tablespoons ground flaxseeds

1 teaspoon salt

1 teaspoon caster sugar

50g (1¾oz) psyllium husk powder

3 tablespoons pumpkin seeds

575ml (1 pint) warm water

7g (¼oz) fast-action dried yeast

2 tablespoons coconut or olive oil, plus extra for brushing

In a large bowl, mix together the buckwheat flour, ground flaxseeds, salt, sugar, psyllium husk powder and 2 tablespoons of the pumpkin seeds. In a large jug, whisk the water with the yeast.

Pour the yeast mixture and oil into the flour mixture and mix well to make a sticky dough.

Tip out the dough on to a lightly floured surface and knead gently for about 10 seconds, then return the dough to the bowl. Cover the bowl with clingfilm and leave in a warm place for 30 minutes to rise.

Line a baking sheet with nonstick baking paper.

Shape the dough into a fat sausage, then brush it with oil and sprinkle over the remaining pumpkin seeds. Transfer the dough to the prepared baking sheet, then cover with a clean tea towel and leave to rise in a warm place for another 30 minutes.

Preheat the oven to 220°C/425°F/Gas Mark 7.

Uncover the dough. Slash the top several times with a sharp knife and sprinkle over a little buckwheat flour. Bake for 35–40 minutes until the loaf is golden brown and sounds hollow when tapped on the base. Leave to cool on a wire rack before slicing.

Spelt sourdough loaf

Makes 1 large loaf

For the starter:
300g (10½oz) stoneground wholegrain spelt flour
350ml (12fl oz) cool or tepid water

For the dough:
400ml (14fl oz) warm water
2 teaspoons caster sugar
150g (5½oz) starter (see above)
500g (1lb 2oz) wholegrain spelt flour, plus extra for dusting
2 teaspoons salt

To make the starter, put 100g (3½oz) of the flour into a plastic container. Add 150ml (¼ pint) of the measured water. Stir well to make a paste. Leave, semi-uncovered, at room temperature for 48 hours.

After this time, small bubbles should have appeared on the surface. Stir in another 100g (3½oz) of the flour and 100ml (3½fl oz) water. Repeat this process 24 hours later. By day 4, your starter should be ready – it will be frothy, with large bubbles.

To make the bread, mix together the warm water and sugar in a large bowl. Add 150g (5½oz) starter and stir until well blended. Mix in the flour and salt to make a sticky, claggy dough. Cover the bowl loosely with clingfilm or a clean tea towel and leave to prove for 1 hour.

With lightly floured hands, stretch and fold the dough in the bowl, then cover loosely and leave to prove for another 30 minutes. Repeat this process twice more, then cover loosely and leave to rise overnight or for about 6 hours, until the dough has doubled in volume.

Tip out the dough on to a floured surface and shape it into a round. Place it in a silicone bread maker or a preheated lidded casserole dish/ Dutch oven (if you just cook it on a baking sheet, the loaf will spread out too much). Leave to prove for a further 30–40 minutes.

Preheat the oven to 220°C/425°F/Gas Mark 7.

Dust the dough with a little flour and make 2 slashes in the top. Bake for 40–45 minutes until the loaf is golden brown and sounds hollow when tapped on the base. If cooking in a casserole dish/Dutch oven, remove the lid for the last 10 minutes of cooking. Leave to cool, then slice.

Tip: You will have some starter left after this recipe. You can use it to make more bread if you keep it alive. To do so, continue to 'feed' it by stirring in flour and water once a week, and store it in the refrigerator.

Sweet French toast with berries & orange yogurt

Serves 4

100g (3½oz) blueberries*
100g (3½oz) strawberries, hulled and quartered
2 oranges
400g (14oz) lactose-free or plant-based low-FODMAP
  yogurt

2 eggs, beaten
50g (1¾oz) caster sugar
2 tablespoons sesame seeds
pinch of ground cinnamon
25g (1oz) unsalted butter or margarine
4 slices of gluten-free low-FODMAP bread

Place the blueberries and strawberries in a bowl. Grate the zest of the oranges and set the zest aside, then segment the oranges, keeping all the juice. Add the orange segments and juice to the bowl with the berries.

Stir the orange zest into the yogurt and chill.

Whisk together the eggs, sugar, sesame seeds and cinnamon.

Melt the butter or margarine in a frying pan over a medium heat. Dip the slices of bread into the egg mixture, then place in the pan and cook for 2–3 minutes on each side until golden.

Serve each slice of French toast topped with fruit and a dollop of the orange-infused yogurt, with the fruit juices poured over the top.

LUNCH

Aubergine toasties with pesto

Serves 4
4 tablespoons extra virgin olive oil
1 large aubergine, sliced lengthways into 1cm (½in) slices
4 slices low-FODMAP gluten-free sourdough bread
2 beef tomatoes, thickly sliced

120g (4¼oz) mozzarella cheese, sliced
salt and black pepper

For the pesto:
50g (1¾oz) basil leaves
1 tablespoon garlic-infused olive oil (see pages 132–3)
55g (2oz) pine nuts
100ml (3½fl oz) extra virgin olive oil
2 tablespoons freshly grated Parmesan cheese

First make the pesto. Put the basil, garlic-infused olive oil, pine nuts, olive oil and salt and pepper in a food processor and process until fairly smooth. Transfer to a bowl, then stir in the Parmesan. Taste and adjust the seasoning if necessary. Set aside until required.

Season the oil with salt and pepper and brush over the aubergine slices. Heat a ridged griddle pan over a medium heat until hot. Add the aubergine slices, working in batches if necessary, and cook for 4–5 minutes on each side until charred and tender. Meanwhile, preheat the grill and use it to toast the sourdough bread to your liking.

Top each piece of toast with an aubergine slice and spread over the pesto. Top with some tomato and mozzarella slices and more pesto. Return to the grill for 1–2 minutes until the cheese is bubbling and golden. Serve straight away.

Cheese, tomato & basil muffins

Makes 8; 1 muffin = 1 portion
oil spray, for oiling
150g (5½oz) gluten-free self-raising flour

½ teaspoon salt

100g (3½oz) polenta

50g (1¾oz) sun-dried tomatoes in oil, drained and chopped*

2 tablespoons chopped basil

65g (2½oz) Cheddar cheese, grated

1 egg, lightly beaten

300ml (½ pint) lactose-free or plant-based milk (such as coconut, hemp, quinoa, rice, almond or hazelnut)

2 tablespoons extra virgin olive oil

butter, to serve

Preheat the oven to 180°C/350°F/Gas Mark 4 and lightly oil 8 holes of a muffin tin with the oil spray.

Sift the flour and salt into a bowl and stir in the polenta, along with the tomatoes, basil and 50g (1¾oz) of the cheese. Make a well in the centre of the mixture.

In a separate bowl or jug, beat together the egg, milk and oil. Pour this mixture into the well and stir together until just combined. The batter should remain a little lumpy.

Divide the batter between the prepared muffin holes and scatter over the remaining cheese. Bake for 20–25 minutes until risen and golden. Leave to cool in the tin for 5 minutes, then transfer to a wire rack to cool. Serve warm, with butter.

Chicken club sandwich

Serves 4

1 tablespoon sunflower oil

4 small boneless, skinless chicken breasts, thinly sliced

8 smoked streaky bacon rashers

12 slices of low-FODMAP gluten-free bread

4 tablespoons light mayonnaise (free from garlic and onion)

125g (4½oz) mozzerella cheese, thinly sliced

4 tomatoes, thinly sliced

40g (1½oz) watercress

Heat the oil in a frying pan over a medium heat. Add the chicken and bacon and fry for 6–8 minutes, turning once or twice, until golden and the chicken is cooked through.

Toast the bread, then spread each slice with mayonnaise on one side. Divide the chicken and bacon between 4 of the pieces of toast, then top each one with some sliced cheese. Add another slice of toast to each one, then top this with the tomato slices and watercress. Complete the sandwich stacks with the final slices of toast.

Press the sandwiches together, then cut each stack into 4 small triangles. Secure with cocktail sticks, if needed, and serve immediately.

Chicken nachos

Makes 4

6 soft wheat-free, low-FODMAP corn tortillas

1 tablespoon sunflower oil

½ teaspoon sea salt flakes

200g (7oz) cooked chicken, chopped

50g (1¾oz) sliced jalapeño peppers from a jar, drained

75g (2¾oz) Cheddar cheese, grated

salt and pepper

150ml (¼ pint) soured cream, to serve

For the salsa:
3 tomatoes, finely chopped
1 red chilli, deseeded and finely chopped
1 tablespoon chopped coriander, plus extra leaves to garnish
juice of 1 lime

Preheat the oven to 190°C/375°F/Gas Mark 5.

Brush the tortillas with the oil then sprinkle with sea salt and cut into triangles. Spread out on 2 baking sheets and bake for 8–10 minutes until crisp. Leave to cool while you make the salsa.

In a bowl, mix together the salsa ingredients and season with salt and pepper.

Sprinkle the cooked chicken over the baked tortillas, along with the jalapeño slices and the salsa. Scatter the grated Cheddar over the top and return to the oven for 3–4 minutes to melt the cheese. Garnish with coriander leaves and serve with soured cream.

Crispy salmon noodle soup

Serves 2
2 teaspoons groundnut oil
2 boneless salmon fillets, skin on
500ml (18fl oz) homemade chicken stock (see page 133)
1 tablespoon lime juice
2 teaspoons fish sauce
1 tablespoon light soy sauce
1.5cm (⅝ inch) piece of fresh root ginger, peeled and cut into matchsticks
1 small red chilli, thinly sliced

2 heads of pak choi, sliced in half lengthways
150g (5½oz) buckwheat soba noodles
coriander leaves, to garnish

Heat the oil in a large frying pan over a medium heat. Add the salmon fillets and fry, skin-side down, for 3–5 minutes until the skin is really crispy. Turn carefully and cook for a further minute on the other side until cooked but still slightly rare. Transfer to a plate and keep warm.

Pour the stock into a saucepan over a medium heat, then add the lime juice, fish sauce, soy sauce and ginger and bring to the boil. Simmer for 3–4 minutes, then add the chilli and pak choi and simmer for another 4–5 minutes until the pak choi is tender.

Meanwhile, cook the noodles in a pan of boiling water for 4–5 minutes, or according to the packet instructions, until just tender. Drain and heap into serving bowls.

Ladle the hot broth over the noodles and top each bowl with a salmon fillet. Serve immediately, garnished with coriander leaves.

Feta, herb & rocket frittata

Serves 2

4 eggs, beaten
2 tablespoons chopped fresh herbs, such as chives, chervil and parsley
1 tablespoon double cream
1 tablespoon olive oil
1 bunch of spring onions (green parts only), sliced
½ red pepper, cored, deseeded and finely sliced
80g (2¾oz) feta cheese

large handful of rocket leaves
salt and black pepper

In a bowl, beat together the eggs, herbs and cream, and season with salt and pepper.

Heat the oil in a nonstick frying pan with a flameproof handle. Add the spring onions and red pepper and cook over a medium heat for 3–4 minutes until just softened.

Pour in the egg mixture and cook for about 3 minutes until almost set, then crumble over the feta. Meanwhile, preheat the grill to high.

Place the pan under the grill and cook for 2–3 minutes until the top of the frittata is golden brown. Top with the rocket and serve.

Fusilli with Parmesan & pine nuts

Serves 4
300g (10½oz) gluten-free fusilli
55g (2oz) pine nuts
75g (2¾oz) butter
2 tablespoons olive oil
handful of basil leaves
75g (2¾oz) Parmesan cheese, grated
salt and pepper

Cook the pasta in a large saucepan of salted boiling water according to the packet instructions until al dente, then drain.

Meanwhile, toast the pine nuts on a grill pan under a medium grill, or in a dry frying pan over a medium heat. Watch them constantly and move them around to make sure they brown evenly.

Melt the butter with the oil in a small saucepan over a low heat.

Return the drained pasta to its pan and stir in half the basil leaves so they start to wilt. Pour over the melted butter and oil, then season with salt and pepper and toss well to combine.

Transfer the pasta to warmed serving plates. Sprinkle with the Parmesan and toasted pine nuts, then scatter over the remaining basil leaves and serve immediately.

Griddled Greek-style sandwiches

Serves 2

6 spring onions (green parts only), chopped
8 cherry tomatoes, quartered
4 pitted black olives, chopped
5cm (2in) piece of cucumber, deseeded and diced
1 teaspoon dried oregano
50g (1¾oz) feta cheese, crumbled
1 teaspoon lemon juice
2 low-FODMAP gluten-free pitta breads
25g (1oz) Cheddar cheese, grated
olive oil, for brushing
black pepper

In a small bowl, mix together the spring onions, tomatoes, olives, cucumber, oregano and feta. Add the lemon juice, then season to taste with pepper and gently stir.

Split open each pitta bread. Divide the feta mixture between the bottom halves of the pitta breads, then scatter over the Cheddar. Cover with the top halves of the pitta breads.

Brush a griddle pan with oil and place over a medium heat. Once the pan is hot, add the sandwiches. Cook for 2–3 minutes on each side, pressing them down gently with a spatula, until they are golden and the cheese is melted. Serve immediately.

Peanut soup

Serves 6

1 tablespoon sunflower oil

1 bunch of spring onions (green parts only), finely chopped

2 carrots, diced

500g (1lb 2oz) tomatoes, skinned if you prefer, chopped

½ teaspoon dried chilli flakes

100g (3½oz) roasted salted peanuts

1 litre (1¾ pints) homemade fish or vegetable stock (see page 133)

salt and pepper

To garnish:

dried chilli flakes

35g (1¼oz) peanuts, roughly chopped

Heat the oil in a saucepan over a medium heat. Add the spring onions and carrots and fry for 5 minutes, stirring until softened and just turning golden around the edges. Stir in the tomatoes and chilli flakes and cook for 1 minute.

Grind the peanuts in a spice mill or high-powered blender until you have a fine powder like ground almonds. Stir this into the tomato mixture, then add the stock and bring to the boil. Reduce the heat to low, then cover and simmer for 30 minutes. Remove half the soup from the pan and mash or purée it until smooth. Return to the pan with the rest of the soup and stir to warm it through. Taste and adjust the seasoning if needed, then ladle the soup into bowls. Garnish with chilli flakes and peanuts and serve.

Potato pizza Margherita

Serves 3–4

1kg (2lb 4oz) baking potatoes, peeled and cut into small chunks

3 tablespoons olive oil, plus extra for oiling

1 egg, beaten

50g (1¾oz) Parmesan or Cheddar cheese, grated

4 tablespoons tomato purée or tomato ketchup (make sure it's free from fructose, onions and garlic)

500g (1lb 2oz) small tomatoes, thinly sliced

125g (4½oz) mozzarella cheese, thinly sliced

1 tablespoon chopped thyme, plus extra sprigs to garnish (optional)

salt

Preheat the oven to 200°C/400°F/Gas Mark 6 and grease a baking sheet with oil. Cook the potatoes in a saucepan of salted boiling water for 15 minutes or until tender. Drain well, then return to the pan and leave to cool for 10 minutes.

Add 2 tablespoons of the oil to the saucepan with the potatoes, then add the egg and half the grated cheese. Mix well, then turn out on to the prepared baking sheet and spread out to form a 25cm (10in) round. Bake for 15 minutes.

Remove from the oven and spread with the tomato purée or ketchup. Arrange the tomato and mozzarella slices on top. Scatter with the remaining cheese, along with the thyme (if using) and a little salt. Drizzle with the remaining oil.

Return to the oven for a further 15 minutes, or until the potato is crisp around the edges and the cheese is melting. Cut into generous wedges, garnish with thyme sprigs, if using, and serve.

Quinoa, feta & raw vegetable salad

Serves 4

50g (1¾oz) quinoa
2 large tomatoes, diced
½ cucumber, diced
small bunch of flat-leaf parsley, chopped
small bunch of mint, chopped
6 spring onions (green parts only), chopped
50g (1¾oz) shredded mangetout
1 red pepper, cored, deseeded and diced
100g (3½oz) feta, crumbled

For the dressing:

3 tablespoons olive oil
1 tablespoon lemon juice
½ teaspoon Dijon mustard

Cook the quinoa in a saucepan of boiling water for 8–9 minutes, or according to the packet instructions, then drain and refresh under cold running water. Meanwhile, in a large bowl, mix together the tomatoes, cucumber, parsley, mint, spring onions, mangetout and pepper.

Whisk together the dressing ingredients in a small bowl or jug.

Stir the cooked quinoa into the bowl with the other salad ingredients. Drizzle over the dressing and top with the crumbled feta. Serve immediately.

Rösti with ham & eggs

Serves 2

500g (1lb 2oz) waxy potatoes, such as Désirée, peeled and grated

25g (1oz) butter

2 eggs

2 slices of smoked ham

salt and black pepper

tomato ketchup, to serve (make sure it's free from fructose, onions and garlic)

Place the grated potatoes on a clean tea towel. Wrap the towel around them, then squeeze to remove the excess moisture. Transfer the grated potatoes to a bowl and season to taste with salt and pepper.

Melt the butter in a large nonstick frying pan over a medium heat. Divide the potato mixture into quarters and form each portion into a 10cm (4in) cake. Add these to the pan and cook for 5–6 minutes on each side until lightly golden.

Meanwhile, poach or fry the eggs to your liking (see page 179 for how to poach an egg).

Serve 2 rösti per person, along with an egg and a slice of smoked ham, and some tomato ketchup on the side.

Salmon fishcakes with dill sauce

Serves 4

450g (1lb) potatoes, peeled and cubed

3 tablespoons olive oil

500g (1lb 2oz) skinless salmon fillets

1 tablespoon chopped dill

finely grated zest of 1 lemon

gluten-free plain flour, for dusting

1 egg, beaten

75g (2¾oz) dried breadcrumbs (made from low-FODMAP
   gluten-free bread)

salt and pepper

green salad, to serve

For the dill sauce:

3 tablespoons mayonnaise (make sure it's free from garlic
   and onions)

3 tablespoons lactose-free or plant-based low-FODMAP
   natural yogurt

handful of dill, chopped

1 cornichon, sliced

Cook the potatoes in a saucepan of lightly salted boiling water for 12 minutes until soft. Drain well and roughly mash.

Meanwhile, rub 1 teaspoon of the oil over the salmon and season well. Preheat the grill to high, then grill the salmon for 10 minutes until cooked through. Leave to cool a little, then break into large flakes.

In a small jug or bowl, mix together the ingredients for the sauce and set aside. In a large bowl, mix together the crushed potatoes, flaked salmon, dill and lemon zest. Lightly wet your hands, then shape the mixture into 8 fishcakes. Dust each fishcake with a little flour. Put the beaten egg in a shallow bowl and the breadcrumbs in another. Dip each fishcake into the egg, followed by the breadcrumbs, making sure they are well coated.

Heat the remaining oil in a large, nonstick frying pan over a medium heat. Cook the fishcakes for 3–4 minutes on each side until golden and crisp. Serve with a green salad and the dill sauce.

Smoked haddock omelettes

Makes 4

150g (5½oz) smoked haddock

125ml (4fl oz) lactose-free or plant-based milk (such as coconut, hemp, quinoa, rice, almond or hazelnut)

12 eggs

50g (1¾oz) butter

200g (7oz) spinach leaves

salt and pepper

Place the haddock and milk in a saucepan over a medium heat and poach the fish for 3–4 minutes, or until cooked. Remove from the pan with a slotted spoon, then remove and discard the skin and any bones. Flake the fish into a bowl.

Beat the eggs in a separate large bowl and season.

Heat a quarter of the butter in a frying pan over a medium heat until foaming, then pour in a quarter of the beaten egg. Stir it a little with a fork, tipping the pan so the egg covers the base, then cook for 3–4 minutes until set.

Place a quarter of the spinach on the omelette, then top with a quarter of the fish. Fold the omelette over and cook for a further minute. Serve on a warm plate.

Repeat the process with the remaining ingredients to make the other three omelettes.

Smoked salmon & prawn sushi

Serves 4-6

450ml (16fl oz) water

250g (9oz) sushi rice

4 tablespoons rice vinegar

1 teaspoon horseradish sauce, plus extra to serve

250g (9oz) cooked tiger prawns, peeled

grated zest and juice of 2 limes

5 sheets of nori seaweed

200g (7oz) sliced smoked salmon

40g (1½oz) pickled sushi ginger, drained

325g (11½oz) jar of red pimentos, drained and cut into
   long strips

6 spring onions (green parts only), cut into long, thin strips

Bring the water to the boil in a saucepan, then add the rice. Reduce the heat to low, then cover and simmer gently for 20–25 minutes until the rice is very soft. Drain off any excess water. In a small bowl, mix together the vinegar and horseradish, then stir this into the rice. Leave to cool.

Toss the prawns in a bowl with the lime zest and juice and set aside.

Place one nori sheet on a bamboo rolling mat. Spoon over a fifth of the rice and spread it in an even layer, leaving a small border of nori showing. Arrange a fifth of the smoked salmon in a long line in the centre of the rice. Next to that add a fifth of the prawns, then top with some ginger, pimentos and spring onions.

Using the rolling mat to help you, roll up the nori sheet so the rice wraps around the filling and the edges of the nori overlap slightly. Rock back and forth to create an even shape. Repeat to make the remaining rolls. Wrap them individually in clingfilm and chill until required.

When you're ready to serve the sushi, cut the rolls into thick slices and arrange on a plate with the cut edges uppermost. Serve with extra horseradish.

Thai beef salad with herbs

Serves 4

4 tablespoons Thai fish sauce
finely grated zest and juice of ½ lime
2 teaspoons caster sugar
1 tablespoon garlic-infused olive oil (see pages 132–3)
1 teaspoon finely grated fresh root ginger
1 lemon grass stalk, finely chopped
1 red chilli, finely chopped
handful of chopped coriander
handful of chopped mint
1 tablespoon vegetable oil
500g (1lb 2oz) steak
250g (9oz) cherry tomatoes, quartered
½ cucumber, thinly sliced
handful of green salad leaves, such as lettuce and
    baby spinach

In a small bowl or jug, mix together the fish sauce, lime zest and juice and sugar. Stir until the sugar dissolves, then add the garlic-infused olive oil, ginger, lemon grass, chilli and herbs to make a dressing.

Rub the vegetable oil over the steak and season to taste. Place a griddle pan over a high heat until smoking hot, then add the steak and cook for 2–3 minutes on each side. Remove from the pan and allow to rest for a couple of minutes before cutting into slices.

Place the tomatoes, cucumber and salad leaves on a serving plate, then arrange the warm beef on top. Drizzle over the dressing and serve immediately.

Asian rice paper rolls

Makes 12
125g (4½oz) cooked peeled prawns
¼ cucumber, cut into matchsticks
handful of coriander, chopped
handful of mint, chopped
handful of Thai basil, chopped
150g (5½oz) cold cooked rice vermicelli
¼ iceberg lettuce, shredded
12 round rice paper sheets
lime wedges, to serve

For the dipping sauce:
2 tablespoons light soy sauce
juice of 1 lime
1 tablespoon Thai fish sauce
1 tablespoon sesame seeds, toasted

In a large bowl, mix together the prawns, cucumber, herbs, vermicelli and lettuce.

Soak 1 rice sheet in a bowl of warm water for 20 seconds, then drain on kitchen paper. Place some prawn mixture on the rice sheet, leaving about 2.5cm (1in) space at the top and the bottom of the sheet. Fold over the top and bottom edges, then roll up the sheet. Repeat with the remaining rice sheets and filling.

Whisk together all the dipping sauce ingredients in a small bowl and serve with the rolls and lime wedges.

Wild rice & griddled chicken salad

Serves 4

2 teaspoons garlic-infused olive oil (see pages 132–3)

1 teaspoon balsamic vinegar

4 small boneless, skinless chicken breasts, halved horizontally

For the rice salad:

200g (7oz) mixed wild and basmati rice

2 red peppers, roasted and sliced

6 spring onions (green parts only), sliced

125g (4½oz) cherry tomatoes, quartered

75g (2¾oz) rocket leaves

75g (2¾oz) soft goats' cheese, crumbled*

For the dressing:

juice of ½ lemon

1 teaspoon Dijon mustard

1 teaspoon maple syrup

2 tablespoons olive oil

In a non-metallic bowl, mix together the garlic-infused olive oil and vinegar. Add the chicken and turn to coat in the marinade. Cover and leave to marinate in the refrigerator for at least 30 minutes.

Meanwhile, cook the rice in a saucepan of boiling water according to the packet instructions. Drain and leave to cool, then mix with the peppers, spring onions, tomatoes, rocket and goats' cheese in a large bowl.

Whisk together the dressing ingredients in a small bowl or jug and stir into the rice salad. Spoon the salad on to 4 serving plates.

Heat a griddle pan over a high heat until hot. Add the chicken and cook for 3–4 minutes on each side until cooked through. Just before serving, slice the griddled chicken and arrange on top of the salad.

DINNER

Aubergine & courgette parmigiana

Serves 6
500ml (18fl oz) passata
handful of basil leaves, torn
4 tablespoons garlic-infused olive oil (see pages 132–3)
450g (1lb) aubergines, cut lengthways into 1cm (½in) slices
390g (13½oz) courgettes, cut lengthways into 1cm (½in) slices
4 red peppers, cored, deseeded and sliced lengthways
180g (6¼oz) mozzarella cheese, chopped
60g (2¼oz) Parmesan cheese, freshly grated
salt and pepper

Preheat the oven to 180°C/350°F/Gas Mark 4.

Combine the passata and basil in a bowl. Season with salt and pepper and stir in half the garlic-infused oil. In another bowl, toss the aubergines, courgettes and peppers in the remaining oil to coat.

Heat a ridged griddle pan over a high heat until smoking hot. Add the vegetables, in batches, and cook for 2–3 minutes on each side until tender all the way through.

Spoon a little of the passata mixture into the base of a deep 30 × 20cm (12 × 8in) baking dish. Cover with a layer of aubergines and courgettes, then scatter with some of the mozzarella. Spoon over 4 tablespoons of the passata mixture and scatter over some Parmesan. Continue layering in this way until all the ingredients are used up, finishing with a layer of passata mixture followed by Parmesan.

Bake for 25–30 minutes, or until golden and bubbly. Serve.

Aubergine, tomato & chilli curry

Serves 4

100ml (3½fl oz) garlic-infused vegetable oil (see pages 132–3)

300g (10½oz) aubergines, sliced into 2cm (¾in) batons

260g (9½oz) courgettes, sliced into 2cm (¾in) batons

2 small red peppers, cored, deseeded and sliced into 2cm (¾in) batons

2 bunches of spring onions (green parts only), sliced

3 teaspoons finely chopped fresh root ginger

2 red chillies, deseeded and thinly sliced

200g (7oz) tinned chopped tomatoes

6 kaffir lime leaves

1 tablespoon kecap manis (sweet soy sauce)

2 tablespoons dark soy sauce

1 teaspoon soft light brown sugar

juice of 1 lime

small handful of chopped coriander leaves

2 tablespoons chopped roasted peanuts

steamed rice or rice noodles, to serve

Reserve 1 tablespoon of the garlic-infused oil, then heat the remaining oil in a large frying pan over a medium heat. Add the aubergines, courgettes and peppers and fry, stirring occasionally, for 5–6 minutes, or until lightly browned. Remove with a slotted spoon and set aside on a plate lined with kitchen paper to drain.

Heat the reserved oil in the pan over a medium heat. Add the spring onions and cook, stirring occasionally, for 6–7 minutes until softened and lightly browned. Add the ginger, chillies, tomatoes and lime leaves and cook for 2–3 minutes, stirring frequently. Return the aubergines, courgettes and peppers to the pan with a splash of water and simmer gently for 2–3 minutes.

Remove from the heat and stir in the kecap manis, soy sauce, sugar, lime juice and chopped coriander. Spoon into warm bowls, sprinkle over the chopped peanuts and serve with steamed rice or rice noodles.

Beef steaks with mozzarella

Serves 4

2 tablespoons garlic-infused olive oil (see pages 132–3)

1 bunch of spring onions (green parts only), sliced

1 courgette, diced

1 yellow pepper, cored, deseeded and diced
1 aubergine, diced
6 plum tomatoes, skinned and diced
10 basil leaves, chopped
2 tablespoons vegetable oil
4 beef steaks
4 thick slices of mozzarella cheese
salt and pepper

Heat the garlic-infused olive oil in a shallow pan over a medium heat. Add the spring onions and sauté until softened. Add the courgette, yellow pepper and aubergine, and cook for a further 5–10 minutes until softened. Add the tomatoes to the pan, along with a little salt and pepper, then add the chopped basil. Allow the mixture to cool, then cover and chill until required.

Preheat the oven to 200°C/400°F/Gas Mark 6.

Heat the vegetable oil in the same pan over a medium heat. Add the steaks and cook for about 2–4 minutes on each side, or according to taste. Season and remove from the pan.

When ready to serve, place the steaks on a baking sheet. Top each one with a quarter of the vegetables and a thick slice of mozzarella. Place in the oven for 10–15 minutes until piping hot and the cheese is melted, then serve immediately.

Cheese roulade with spinach & walnuts

Serves 4
30g (1oz) unsalted butter
30g (1oz) gluten-free plain flour

200ml (7fl oz) lactose-free or plant-based milk (such as
   coconut, hemp, quinoa, rice, almond or hazelnut)
pinch of cayenne pepper
4 large eggs, separated
2 teaspoons Dijon mustard
40g (1½oz) Cheddar cheese, grated
50g (1¾oz) walnuts, finely chopped
160g (5¾oz) cream cheese
100g (3½oz) baby spinach leaves
3 spring onions (green parts only), finely sliced
salt and pepper

Preheat the oven to 200°C/400°F/Gas Mark 6. Melt the butter in a small saucepan over a medium heat. Grease a 33 × 23cm (13 × 9in) Swiss roll tin with a little of the melted butter, then line it with baking paper.

With the saucepan still on the heat, stir the flour into the remaining melted butter to make a roux. Gradually whisk in the milk and continue to cook until the sauce comes to the boil and is thick and creamy. Remove from the heat, then add the cayenne and season. Stir in the egg yolks, mustard, Cheddar and 40g (1½oz) of the walnuts.

In a large, clean bowl, whisk the egg whites with a hand-held electric whisk until stiff peaks form. Fold the egg whites into the cheese mixture, then gently pour into the prepared tin. Bake for 10–12 minutes until firm to the touch.

Sprinkle the remaining walnuts on to a piece of baking paper slightly larger than the tin. Turn the roulade out of the tin on to the prepared paper and peel off the lining paper from the base of the tin. Use the large piece of baking paper to gently roll up the roulade. Cover with a damp cloth and leave to cool slightly.

Unroll the roulade. Spread it with the cream cheese and sprinkle over the spinach and spring onions, then re-roll, this time without the baking paper. Serve warm or cold.

Chicken & chorizo jambalaya with peppers

Serves 4

175g (6oz) long-grain rice

1 tablespoon olive oil

225g (8oz) piece of chorizo sausage (make sure it's free from garlic), cut into chunky slices

1 bunch of spring onions (green parts only), chopped

375g (13oz) boneless, skinless chicken breasts, cut into chunks

2 red peppers, cored, deseeded and cut into chunks

1 yellow pepper, cored, deseeded and cut into chunks

1 celery stick, chopped

2 tablespoons cold water

1 tablespoon cornflour

600ml (20fl oz) homemade chicken stock (see page 133)

400g (14oz) can chopped tomatoes

salt and pepper

4 tablespoons chopped flat-leaf parsley, to serve

Bring a saucepan of lightly salted water to the boil and cook the rice for 15 minutes until tender, then drain.

Meanwhile, heat the oil in a large, heavy-based frying pan and cook the chorizo, spring onions and chicken over a medium heat, stirring occasionally, for 10 minutes until browned and cooked through. Add the peppers and celery and cook, stirring occasionally, for a further 5 minutes.

Blend the measured water with the cornflour to make a slurry, then stir this into the stock. Pour this mixture into the frying pan, along with the tomatoes and bring to the boil. Reduce the heat to low and simmer for 5 minutes before adding the cooked rice. Season generously with pepper.

Serve garnished with the parsley, accompanied by crusty gluten-free low-FODMAP bread and salad, if you like.

Chicken fusilli with red pepper & almond pesto

Serves 4
400g (14oz) gluten-free fusilli
2 shop-bought plain roasted chicken breasts, about 150g (5½oz) each
salt

For the pesto:
5 tablespoons extra virgin olive oil
2 red peppers
large handful of basil leaves, plus extra to garnish
25g (1oz) toasted almonds
25g (1oz) Pecorino cheese, grated, plus extra to serve

To make the pesto, preheat the grill to high. Rub about 1 tablespoon of the olive oil over the red peppers and grill, whole, for 10 minutes, turning often, until charred all over. Place in a plastic food bag, seal and leave for 5 minutes. Once cooled enough to touch, peel off the blackened skin. Cut the peppers in half and remove the seeds.

Place the roasted peppers in a food processor or blender, along with the remaining olive oil, basil, almonds and Pecorino. Whizz to form a thick but smooth paste. Add a little more oil or a drizzle of water if needed. Season well with salt.

Meanwhile, cook the pasta in a large saucepan of salted boiling water according to the packet instructions until al dente. Drain, reserving a little of the cooking water, and return the pasta to the pan. Stir in the pesto, adding a little cooking water to loosen, until the pasta is coated.

Tear the cooked chicken into strips and stir it through the pasta. Serve in bowls, sprinkled with a little extra chopped basil and some grated Pecorino.

Classic bolognese

Serves 4

25g (1oz) unsalted butter

1 tablespoon olive oil

1 small bunch of spring onions (green parts only), finely chopped

1 celery stick, finely chopped

1 carrot, finely chopped

1 bay leaf

200g (7oz) lean minced beef

200g (7oz) lean minced pork

150ml (¼ pint) dry white wine

150ml (¼ pint) lactose-free or plant-based milk (such as coconut, hemp, quinoa, rice, almond or hazelnut)

large pinch of freshly grated nutmeg

2 × 400g (14oz) cans chopped tomatoes

400–600ml (14–20fl oz) homemade chicken stock (see page 133)

400g (14oz) gluten-free fettuccine

salt and black pepper

freshly grated Parmesan cheese, to serve

Melt the butter with the oil in a large, heavy-based saucepan over a low heat. Add the spring onions, celery, carrot and bay leaf and cook, stirring occasionally, for 10 minutes until softened but not coloured. Increase the heat to medium and add the meat. Season with salt and pepper and cook, stirring, until no longer pink.

Pour in the wine and bring to the boil, then reduce the heat to low and simmer gently for 15 minutes until evaporated. Stir in the milk and nutmeg and simmer for a further 15 minutes until the milk has evaporated. Reduce the heat to very low and stir in the tomatoes. Cook, uncovered, for 3–5 hours. The sauce will be very thick, so when it begins to stick, add the stock as needed, 100ml (3½fl oz) at a time.

Cook the pasta in a large saucepan of salted boiling water according to the packet instructions until al dente. Drain thoroughly, reserving a ladleful of the cooking water.

Return the pasta to the pan and place over a low heat. Add the bolognese sauce and stir for 30 seconds, then pour in the reserved pasta cooking water and stir well until the pasta is well coated and looks silky. Serve immediately with a scattering of grated Parmesan.

Comforting fish pie

Serves 4 | Moderate-FODMAP recipe

750g (1lb 10oz) floury potatoes, cut into chunks

2 eggs (optional)

400ml (14fl oz) lactose-free or plant-based milk (such as coconut, hemp, quinoa, rice, almond or hazelnut)

50g (1¾oz) gluten-free plain flour

100g (3½oz) butter

2 tablespoons chopped flat-leaf parsley

25g (1oz) watercress, roughly chopped (optional)

390g (13½oz) shop-bought fish pie mixture (available from the chilled section of supermarkets), or use bite-sized chunks of salmon, white fish fillet and smoked haddock

200g (7oz) raw peeled king prawns

3 tablespoons crème fraîche* (check individual brand against your low-FODMAP app as not all are suitable)

75g (2¾oz) Cheddar cheese, grated

salt and pepper

green salad leaves (such as lettuce and baby spinach), to serve

Preheat the oven to 220°C/425°F/Gas Mark 7.

Cook the potatoes in a pan of lightly salted boiling water for 10–12 minutes until tender.

Meanwhile, hard-boil the eggs (if using) in a pan of simmering water for about 8 minutes. Drain and place under cold running water. Once cool enough to handle, remove the shells and cut the eggs into wedges. Set aside.

Place the milk, flour and half the butter in a saucepan and bring slowly to the boil, stirring constantly with a balloon whisk, until thick and smooth. Simmer for 1–2 minutes, then season lightly and take off the heat.

Stir the parsley, watercress (if using), fish, prawns and eggs into the sauce, then transfer to an ovenproof dish.

Drain the potatoes and mash them with the crème fraîche and the remaining butter. Season to taste, then spoon the mash over the fish mixture and scatter the grated cheese on top. Bake the pie for 12–15 minutes, or until golden and bubbling and the fish is cooked. Serve with a green salad.

Feta & roast vegetable tart

Serves 6

125g (4½oz) gluten-free self-raising flour, plus extra
   for dusting

50g (1¾oz) oatmeal

75g (2¾oz) chilled butter, diced

about 2 tablespoons cold water

1 aubergine, sliced

1 red pepper, cored, deseeded and sliced into thick strips

1 bunch of spring onions (green parts only), sliced

2 courgettes, sliced into batons

3 tomatoes, halved

3 tablespoons garlic-infused olive oil (see pages 132–3)

2 teaspoons chopped fresh rosemary

125g (4½oz) feta cheese, crumbled

2 tablespoons freshly grated Parmesan cheese

salt and pepper

Preheat the oven to 190°C/375°F/Gas Mark 5.

In a bowl, mix together the flour and oatmeal, then add the butter and rub it in until the mixture resembles fine breadcrumbs. Add the water and mix to create a firm dough. Turn out on to a lightly floured surface and knead briefly.

Roll out the pastry and use it to line a 23cm (9in) fluted flan tin, pressing it evenly into the sides. Prick the base with a fork and chill for 15 minutes, then line with nonstick baking paper and add macaroni or baking beans. Bake blind for 10–15 minutes, then remove the paper and macaroni or beans and return to the oven for a further 5 minutes.

Remove the baked pastry case from the oven and increase the temperature to 200°C/400°F/Gas Mark 6.

Mix the vegetables together in a roasting tin. Add the garlic-infused olive oil and rosemary and toss to coat the vegetables evenly. Season to taste. Roast for 35 minutes, or until the vegetables are tender.

Fill the pastry case with the cooked vegetables, then scatter the feta over the top and sprinkle with the Parmesan. Return the tart to the oven for 10 minutes to finish. Serve warm or cold.

Griddled swordfish with salsa verde

Serves 4

1½ teaspoons Dijon mustard
450ml (16fl oz) extra virgin olive oil
4 anchovy fillets, chopped
handful each of fresh flat-leaf parsley, basil, mint and
    tarragon, chopped

2 tablespoons capers, chopped

2 tablespoons garlic-infused olive oil (see pages 132–3)

4 swordfish steaks, about 150g (5½oz) each

juice of 1 lemon

salt and pepper

green salad leaves (such as lettuce and baby spinach),
    to serve

In a bowl, whisk together the mustard and 250ml (9fl oz) of the extra virgin olive oil until they have emulsified. Stir in the anchovies.

Add the herbs and capers to the oil mixture. Gradually add more of the extra virgin olive oil, whisking between each addition, until the sauce has a spooning consistency.

Heat a griddle pan over a medium heat until hot. Brush the swordfish steaks on each side with the garlic-infused olive oil and season well. Griddle for 2–3 minutes on each side, or until cooked through but still very moist.

Add the lemon juice to the salsa verde and spoon it over the griddled fish. Serve with a crisp green salad.

Homemade fish fingers

Serves 4

3 tablespoons gluten-free plain flour

1 large egg, beaten

30g (1oz) breadcrumbs, made from low-FODMAP
    gluten-free bread

25g (1oz) polenta

500g (1lb 2oz) cod fillet, cut into 8 thick pieces

3 tablespoons sunflower oil

200g (7oz) green beans

2 tablespoons butter or olive oil

4 eggs

salt

Place the flour and the beaten egg in two separate shallow bowls, then mix the breadcrumbs and polenta together in a third bowl.

Gently toss the pieces of fish first in the flour, then in the egg and finally in the breadcrumb and polenta mixture to coat.

Heat the sunflower oil in a frying pan over a medium heat and cook the fish fingers carefully for 5–6 minutes, turning occasionally, until golden.

Meanwhile, cook the beans in salted boiling water for 3–5 minutes.

Heat the butter or olive oil in another frying pan and fry the eggs to your liking.

Drain the beans and serve with the fish fingers and fried eggs.

Horseradish beef with quinoa

Serves 4

625g (1lb 6oz) beef fillet, rolled and tied

1 tablespoon creamed horseradish

2 tablespoons olive oil

300g (10½oz) quinoa

1 small bunch of spring onions (green parts only), finely sliced

125g (4½oz) oyster mushrooms, sliced

1 tablespoon chopped flat-leaf parsley

1 tablespoon chopped mint

40g (1½oz) rocket leaves

3 tablespoons balsamic glaze

Preheat the oven to 200°C/400°F/Gas Mark 6.

Brush the beef with the horseradish. Heat 1 tablespoon of the oil in a frying pan over a high heat, then add the beef and sear on all sides until browned. Transfer to a roasting tin and roast for 20 minutes. Cover with foil and leave to rest for 5–6 minutes, then slice.

While the beef is roasting, cook the quinoa in a saucepan of boiling water for 8–9 minutes, or according to the packet instructions, then drain.

Meanwhile, heat the remaining oil in a large frying pan. Add the spring onions and cook for 2 minutes, then add the mushrooms and cook for a further 5–6 minutes until softened. Remove from the heat and stir in the chopped herbs.

Drain the quinoa and stir into the mushroom mixture. Divide between 4 warm plates and top with the rocket and sliced beef. Serve drizzled with the balsamic glaze.

Italian chicken with tomato sauce

Serves 4

4 chicken legs, halved through the joints

4 tablespoons garlic-infused olive oil (see pages 132–3)

1 large bunch of spring onions (green parts only), finely chopped

75g (2¾oz) pancetta, diced

3 bay leaves

4 tablespoons dry vermouth or white wine

2 × 400g (14oz) cans chopped tomatoes

1 teaspoon caster sugar

3 tablespoons tomato purée

25g (1oz) basil leaves, torn into pieces

8 black olives, pitted

salt and pepper

Season the chicken pieces with salt and pepper. Heat the oil in a large saucepan or sauté pan over a medium heat and fry the chicken on all sides until browned. Transfer to a plate and set aside.

Add the spring onions and pancetta to the pan and fry gently for 10 minutes. Add the bay leaves and fry for a further 1 minute.

Add the vermouth or wine, along with the tomatoes, sugar, tomato purée and seasoning and bring to the boil. Return the chicken pieces to the pan and reduce the heat to its lowest setting. Cook very gently, uncovered, for about 1 hour or until the chicken is very tender.

Stir in the basil and olives and check the seasoning before serving.

Prawn & coconut curry

Serves 4

1 teaspoon cumin seeds

3 cardamom pods

2 bunches of spring onions (green parts only), sliced

4 tablespoons garlic-infused vegetable oil (see pages 132–3)

1 bay leaf

6 curry leaves

2cm (¾in) piece of fresh root ginger, peeled and chopped

½ teaspoon ground turmeric

½ teaspoon asafoetida

1 red chilli, deseeded and chopped

200ml (7fl oz) coconut milk

125g (4½oz) tomatoes, halved

150ml (¼ pint) water

400g (14oz) raw prawns, peeled

1 tablespoon butter

fresh coriander leaves, chopped

steamed rice, to serve

Put the cumin and cardamom in a small dry frying pan and cook for 30 seconds until aromatic. Remove from the heat and set aside.

Place the spring onions in a food processor with 2 tablespoons of the oil and whizz until smooth.

Heat the remaining oil in a pan over a medium heat. Add the spring onion paste, bay leaf and curry leaves and cook for 7–10 minutes until light brown.

Meanwhile, whizz the ginger in a small food processor until smooth. Add to the pan, along with the toasted spices and the turmeric, asafoetida, chilli, coconut milk, tomatoes and water. Simmer for 5 minutes, then add the prawns and cook for 3 minutes until cooked through. Stir in the butter until melted. Scatter over the coriander leaves and serve with steamed rice.

Moorish pork skewers

Serves 4-6

2 teaspoons cumin seeds

2 teaspoons coriander seeds

2 teaspoons fennel seeds

1 teaspoon sweet smoked paprika

squeeze of lemon juice

3 tablespoons garlic-infused olive oil (see pages 132–3)

handful of flat-leaf parsley, chopped, plus extra to garnish

500g (1lb 2oz) pork fillet, cubed

salt and pepper

Place the cumin, coriander and fennel seeds in a spice grinder and crush to a fine powder. Alternatively, use a pestle and mortar. Tip into a bowl and mix with the paprika, lemon juice, garlic-infused olive oil and parsley, then season with salt and pepper. Add the pork to the bowl and stir until well coated. Cover and leave to marinate in the refrigerator for at least 2 hours or preferably overnight.

Thread the pork on to metal skewers. Heat a griddle pan over a high heat until smoking hot, then add the skewers and cook for 10 minutes, turning frequently, until charred and just cooked through. Serve immediately, scattered with extra parsley.

Pad Thai

Serves 2

250g (9oz) dried rice noodles

1½ tablespoons kecap manis (sweet soy sauce)

1½ tablespoons lime juice

1 tablespoon Thai fish sauce

½ teaspoon asafoetida

1 tablespoon water

3 tablespoons groundnut oil

1 bunch of spring onions (green parts only), sliced

1 small red chilli, deseeded and chopped

125g (4½oz) firm tofu, diced

2 eggs, lightly beaten

125g (4½oz) bean sprouts

1 tablespoon chopped coriander

4 tablespoons salted peanuts, chopped

Cook the noodles in boiling water for 5 minutes until softened. Drain and immediately refresh under cold water, then drain again and set aside.

In a small bowl, combine the soy sauce, lime juice, fish sauce, asafoetida and measured water, then set aside.

Heat the oil in a wok or large frying pan over a medium heat. Add the spring onions and chilli and stir-fry for 30 seconds, then add the noodles and tofu and stir-fry for 2–3 minutes until heated through.

Carefully push the noodle mixture to the sides of the pan, clearing the centre of the pan. Add the eggs to the centre and heat gently for 1 minute without stirring, then gently start 'scrambling' the eggs with a spoon. Bring the noodles back into the centre and stir well until combined with the eggs.

Add the soy sauce mixture and cook for 1 minute, or until heated through. Stir in the bean sprouts and coriander. Spoon into bowls and serve immediately, topped with the peanuts.

Prawn, tomato & feta rigatoni

Serves 4

2 tablespoons garlic-infused olive oil (see pages 132-3)

1 bunch of spring onions (green parts only), finely chopped

1 teaspoon tomato purée

juice of ½ lemon

1 teaspoon caster sugar

½ teaspoon dried chilli flakes

400g (14oz) can chopped tomatoes

200g (7oz) frozen large raw peeled prawns

400g (14oz) gluten-free rigatoni

50g (1¾oz) feta cheese

salt and pepper

chopped flat-leaf parsley, to garnish

Heat the oil in a saucepan over a medium heat, then add the spring onions and cook for a couple of minutes until softened. Stir in the tomato purée, then add the lemon juice, sugar, chilli flakes and tomatoes. Bring to the boil, then reduce the heat to low and simmer for 10 minutes.

Remove the pan from the heat then, using a stick blender, whizz the contents to a smooth purée. Return to the heat and add the prawns. Cook for 3–5 minutes, or until they have turned pink and are just cooked through. Season well.

Meanwhile, cook the pasta in a large saucepan of salted boiling water according to the packet instructions until al dente. Drain, reserving a little of the cooking water, then add the pasta to the pan with the prawn sauce and stir, adding a little of the cooking water if needed. Spoon into serving bowls, then crumble over the feta and serve sprinkled with the parsley.

Roasted chicken thighs with root vegetables & maple syrup

Serves 4

4 chicken thighs

300g (10½oz) parsnips, quartered lengthways

5 large carrots, peeled and quartered lengthways

3 tablespoons olive oil

3 tablespoons maple syrup

pepper

4 tablespoons chopped flat-leaf parsley, to garnish

mashed potatoes and steamed leafy greens, such as
   spinach, collard greens or chard, to serve (optional)

Preheat the oven to 220°C/425°F/Gas Mark 7.

Put the chicken in a roasting tin with the vegetables. Drizzle over the oil and shake the vegetables and chicken to coat. Season with pepper and roast for 20–25 minutes, or until golden, drizzling over the maple syrup for the final 3 minutes of cooking. Scatter over the parsley and serve with mashed potatoes and steamed leafy greens, if liked.

Roast herbed pork belly

Serves 4–6

10 sage leaves, roughly chopped

2 large rosemary sprigs, roughly chopped

1 tablespoon fennel seeds

4 tablespoons garlic-infused olive oil (see pages 132–3)

1 boned pork belly joint, about 1.25kg (2lb 12oz)

salt and pepper

roast potatoes and steamed leafy greens, such as spinach, collard greens or chard, to serve (optional)

Preheat the oven to 220°C/425°F/Gas Mark 7.

In a small bowl, mix together the sage, rosemary, fennel seeds and half the oil.

Place the pork on a chopping board, skin-side up, and score the rind at 2.5cm (1in) intervals (the easiest way of doing this is with a Stanley knife). Turn the meat over, skin-side down, and season with salt and pepper. Rub the herb mixture all over the flesh. Roll the pork up with the skin on the outside and tie it tightly with string. Rub the skin all over with the remaining oil and a generous amount of salt.

Roast for 20 minutes, then reduce the oven temperature to 160°C/325°F/Gas Mark 3 and roast for a further 1½ hours. Leave the meat to rest for 10 minutes before carving. Serve with roast potatoes and steamed leafy greens, if liked.

Seafood stir-fry

Serves 4

2 teaspoons brown sugar

grated zest and juice of 1 lime

2 tablespoons tamari soy sauce

24 raw peeled tiger or jumbo king prawns

50g (1¾oz) squid rings

125g (4½oz) mussels, shelled

150g (5½oz) ribbon rice noodles

1 tablespoon vegetable oil

1 teaspoon sesame oil

1 bunch of spring onions (green parts only), sliced

1 red pepper, cored, deseeded and sliced

150g (5½oz) bean sprouts

150g (5½oz) pak choi, chopped

In a small jug or bowl, mix together the sugar, lime zest and juice and tamari. Place the prawns, squid and mussels in a bowl, then pour over the marinade and leave for 5 minutes.

Meanwhile, cook the noodles in a pan of boiling water according to the packet instructions. Drain and refresh under cold water.

Heat the vegetable and sesame oils in a wok over a high heat. Add the seafood and stir-fry for 2–3 minutes until the prawns have turned pink. Remove from the wok and set aside on a plate.

Add the spring onions and red pepper to the wok and stir-fry for 2 minutes, then add the bean sprouts and pak choi and stir-fry for a further 1–2 minutes. Return the seafood to the pan, along with the drained rice noodles, and stir-fry for 2–3 minutes. Serve immediately.

Shepherd's pie

Serves 4–6

1 tablespoon olive oil

1 bunch of spring onions (green parts only), finely chopped

1 carrot, peeled and diced

1 tablespoon chopped thyme

500g (1lb 2oz) minced lamb

400g (14oz) can chopped tomatoes

4 tablespoons tomato purée

750g (1lb 10oz) potatoes, such as Désirée, peeled and cubed

50g (1¾oz) butter

3 tablespoons lactose-free or plant-based milk (such as coconut, hemp, quinoa, rice, almond or hazelnut)

75g (2¾oz) Cheddar cheese, grated

salt and black pepper

Preheat the oven to 190°C/375°F/Gas Mark 5.

Heat the oil in a saucepan over a low heat. Add the spring onions, carrot and thyme and cook gently for 10 minutes until soft and golden.

Add the minced lamb and increase the heat to high, breaking up the lamb with a wooden spoon. Cook for 5 minutes until browned. Add the tomatoes, tomato purée and salt and pepper to taste. Bring to the boil, then reduce the heat to low, cover and simmer for 30 minutes.

Remove the lid and cook for a further 15 minutes until thickened.

Meanwhile, put the potatoes in a large saucepan of lightly salted water and bring to the boil. Reduce the heat and simmer for 15–20 minutes until really tender. Drain well and return to the pan. Mash in the butter, milk and half the cheese and season to taste with salt and pepper.

Spoon the minced lamb mixture into a 2-litre (3½-pint) baking dish and carefully spoon the mash over the top, spreading over the surface of the filling. Use a fork to make lines in the top of the mash, then scatter over the remaining cheese. Bake for 20–25 minutes until bubbling and golden, then serve.

Pepper & tomato paella with pine nuts

Serves 4

3 tablespoons olive oil

2 red peppers, cored, deseeded and thinly sliced

1 yellow pepper, cored, deseeded and thinly sliced

1 small bunch of spring onions (green parts only), sliced

225g (8oz) paella rice

1.2 litres (2 pints) homemade vegetable stock (see page 133)

175g (6oz) plum tomatoes on the vine, halved

3 tablespoons lightly toasted pine nuts

3 tablespoons chopped flat-leaf parsley

salt

Heat 2 tablespoons of the oil in a large, heavy-based frying pan over a medium heat. Add the peppers and spring onions and cook for 4–5 minutes until softened.

Add the rice and stir well, then season with some salt. Pour in the vegetable stock and bring to the boil, then cover and simmer for 20 minutes until the stock is almost all absorbed and the rice is tender and cooked through.

Meanwhile, heat the remaining oil in a separate frying pan over a medium heat. Add the vine tomatoes and cook for 2–3 minutes on each side until softened.

Add the tomatoes to the rice and gently toss through. Remove from the heat and scatter with the pine nuts and flat-leaf parsley, then serve.

DESSERTS & SWEET TREATS

Banana & maple syrup flapjacks

Serves 4

oil, for greasing

25g (1oz) light muscovado sugar

175g (6oz) unsalted butter

2½ tablespoons maple syrup

1 large firm and unripe banana, mashed

300g (10½oz) rolled oats

75g (2¾oz) dried banana chips, roughly broken

Preheat the oven to 180°C/350°F/Gas Mark 4 and lightly grease a 22cm (8½ inch) square cake tin.

Place the sugar, butter and maple syrup in a saucepan over a medium heat and heat, stirring occasionally, until the butter has melted and the sugar dissolved. Remove from the heat.

Stir in the mashed banana and oats and mix well.

Spoon half of the oat mixture into the prepared tin, then sprinkle over the banana chips and top with the remaining oat mixture. Press down and level the top.

Bake for 20–22 minutes until golden. Remove from the oven and cut into 12 bars while still hot. Leave to cool in the tin. The flapjacks will keep in an airtight container for up to 4 days.

Chewy nutty chocolate brownies

Makes 15

75g (2¾oz) gluten-free dark chocolate, broken into pieces

100g (3½oz) unsalted butter, plus extra for greasing

200g (7oz) soft light brown sugar

2 eggs, beaten

few drops of vanilla extract

50g (1¾oz) ground almonds*

25g (1oz) brown rice flour

150g (5½oz) mixed low-FODMAP nuts (such as peanuts, walnuts and macadamia nuts), toasted and roughly chopped

Preheat the oven to 180°C/350°F/Gas Mark 4 and grease and line a 28 × 18cm (11 × 7 inch) baking tin.

Place the chocolate and butter in a large heatproof bowl over a saucepan of simmering water and leave to melt. Once melted, stir in all the remaining ingredients and combine well.

Pour the mixture into the prepared tin and bake for 30 minutes until slightly springy in the centre. Remove from the oven and leave to cool for 10 minutes in the tin, then cut into 15 squares.

The brownies will keep in an airtight container for up to 3 days.

Banana fritters & cinnamon sugar

Serves 4 | Moderate-FODMAP recipe

225g (8oz) gluten-free plain flour

½ teaspoon ground nutmeg

2 teaspoons ground cinnamon

375ml (13fl oz) sparkling water

sunflower oil, for deep-frying

4 firm and unripe bananas, halved lengthways and
 widthways

3 tablespoons demerara sugar

1 tablespoon caster sugar

In a large bowl, mix together the flour, nutmeg and 1 teaspoon of the cinnamon. Make a well in the centre. Gradually add and whisk in enough of the sparkling water to make a smooth batter thick enough to coat the back of a spoon. Leave to stand for 20 minutes.

Fill a deep-sided saucepan a third full with oil and place over a high heat. Heat to 180–190°C (350–375°F), or until a cube of bread browns in 30 seconds. Working in batches, use a pair of tongs to dip the banana pieces into the batter, then gently lower into the hot oil and cook for 30 seconds–1 minute until golden and crisp. Take care not to overcrowd the pan with too many at a time, as they will stick together and the oil temperature will drop. Remove from the pan with a slotted spoon and drain on kitchen paper.

In a small bowl, mix the sugars with the remaining cinnamon, then scatter over the hot fritters and serve.

Blueberry meringue roulade

Serves 8

4 egg whites

250g (9oz) caster sugar, plus extra for sprinkling

1 teaspoon white wine vinegar

1 teaspoon cornflour

For the filling:
grated zest of 1 lime
300ml (½ pint) double cream, whipped
150g (5½oz) blueberries*
3 passion fruit, halved

Preheat the oven to 190°C/375°F/Gas Mark 5 and line a 33 × 23cm (13 × 9 inch) Swiss roll tin with nonstick baking paper, using enough baking paper so that it extends a little above the sides of the tin.

Whisk the egg whites in a large clean bowl until stiff. Gradually whisk in the sugar, a teaspoonful at a time, until it has all been added. Whisk for a few minutes more until the meringue mixture is thick and glossy.

Combine the vinegar and cornflour in a small bowl, then whisk into the meringue mixture. Spoon into the prepared tin and spread out until the surface is level. Bake for 10 minutes until biscuit-coloured and well risen, then reduce the oven temperature to 160°C/325°F/Gas Mark 3 and bake for a further 5 minutes until just firm to the touch and the top is slightly cracked.

Meanwhile, cover a clean tea towel with nonstick baking paper and sprinkle with a little caster sugar. Turn out the meringue on to the paper and remove the tin. Leave to cool for 1–2 hours, then carefully peel off the lining paper that was in the tin.

Fold the lime zest into the whipped cream. Spread it over the meringue, then sprinkle with the blueberries and passion fruit seeds. Starting with one of the short sides and using the paper to help, roll up the meringue to form a log. Chill until ready to serve and serve the same day.

Chocolate pots

Serves 6–8

250ml (9fl oz) double cream

75g (2¾oz) caster sugar

200g (7oz) dark chocolate, chopped

2 egg yolks

grated zest of 1 orange

Place the double cream and sugar in a pan over a medium heat and bring to the boil, stirring a few times to melt the sugar.

Place the chocolate, egg yolks and orange zest in a food processor. With the food processor running, pour in the hot cream and whizz until the chocolate melts. Spoon into 4 glasses and serve.

Peanut butter brownle cupcakes

Makes 12

100g (3½oz) unsalted butter

150g (5½oz) dark chocolate

75g (2¾oz) crunchy peanut butter

2 large eggs

125g (4½oz) golden caster sugar

75g (2¾oz) gluten-free self-raising flour

50g (1¾oz) dark chocolate chips

Preheat the oven to 200°C/400°F/Gas Mark 6. Line a 12-hole cupcake tin with paper cases. Place the butter, dark chocolate and peanut butter in a saucepan over a medium heat and stir for a few minutes until melted. Meanwhile, in a bowl, whisk together the eggs and sugar.

Stir the melted chocolate mixture and flour into the egg mixture. Carefully spoon the batter into the paper cases, then scatter over the chocolate chips.

Bake the cupcakes for 10–12 minutes until almost firm to the touch. Remove from the oven and leave to cool on a wire rack before serving.

Chocolate raspberry cake

Serves 6–8
sunflower oil, for greasing
8 eggs, separated
pinch of salt
400g (14oz) dark chocolate
150g (5½oz) unsalted butter
50g (1¾oz) caster sugar
225g (8oz) crème fraîche* (check individual brand against your low-FODMAP app as not all are suitable)
grated zest of 1 orange
375g (13oz) raspberries
icing sugar, for dusting

Preheat the oven to 180°C/350°F/Gas Mark 4 and grease 2 × 18cm (7 inch) round cake tins.

In a small bowl, whisk the egg yolks with the salt.

Melt the chocolate and butter in a heatproof bowl set over a saucepan of gently simmering water. Leave the melted chocolate to cool for 2–3 minutes, then fold in the egg yolks.

In a clean, grease-free bowl, whisk the egg whites until stiff peaks form, then gradually whisk in the sugar.

Fold the egg whites into the chocolate mixture and pour into the prepared tins. Bake for 15 minutes, then remove from the tins and leave to cool.

Meanwhile, mix together the crème fraîche and orange zest.

Spread the orange cream over one of the cakes and top with half of the raspberries. Place the other cake on top and decorate with the remaining raspberries. Dust with icing sugar to serve.

Coconut rice pudding brûlée

Serves 4 | Moderate-FODMAP recipe
75g (2¾oz) Thai fragrant rice or pudding rice
50g (1¾oz) caster sugar
400ml (14fl oz) can coconut milk*
4 tablespoons demerara sugar
rhubarb compote, to serve

Put the rice in a saucepan with the sugar and coconut milk. Refill the coconut milk can with water and add to the pan.

Place over a medium heat and bring the mixture to the boil, stirring, then reduce the heat to low and leave to simmer, stirring occasionally, for 20 minutes until the rice is tender and the liquid is absorbed.

Spoon the mixture into individual heatproof dishes, level the surface and leave to cool. Chill for 2–3 hours or overnight.

Just before serving, sprinkle 1 tablespoon of the demerara sugar evenly over the surface of each dish. Place under a hot grill or use a cook's blowtorch to melt and caramelize the sugar.

Leave to cool for 10 minutes to harden the caramel before serving with rhubarb compote.

Cranberry, oat & raisin cookies

Makes 12; 1 cookie = 1 portion

50g (1¾oz) unsalted butter

6 tablespoons maple syrup

125g (4½oz) gluten-free wholemeal plain flour

75g (2¾oz) rolled oats

1 teaspoon gluten-free baking powder

½ teaspoon ground cinnamon

½ teaspoon ground ginger

pinch of freshly grated nutmeg

50g (1¾oz) dried cranberries*

50g (1¾oz) raisins

Preheat the oven to 180°C/350°F/Gas Mark 4 and line a large baking sheet with baking paper.

Heat the butter with the maple syrup in a saucepan over a low heat, stirring, until melted. Remove from the heat, then add the remaining ingredients and mix well.

Spoon the mixture on to the prepared baking sheet in 12 large mounds and press each down slightly with the back of a spoon. Bake for 8–10 minutes until the edges are golden but the centres still soft.

Leave the cookies to cool for 2–3 minutes on the baking sheet before transferring to a wire rack to cool completely.

The cookies will keep in an airtight container for up to 3 days.

Giant choc chip & orange cookies

Makes 12

125g (4½oz) soft light brown sugar

125g (4½oz) granulated sugar

150g (5½oz) unsalted butter, softened

2 teaspoons finely grated orange zest

1 large egg, lightly beaten

1 teaspoon vanilla extract

250g (9oz) gluten-free plain flour

1 teaspoon gluten free baking powder

150g (5½oz) good-quality dark chocolate with orange,
   roughly chopped into chunks

Place the sugars, butter and orange zest in a large bowl and beat with a hand-held electric whisk until smooth and pale. Add the beaten egg and vanilla extract and beat until combined.

Sift in the flour and baking powder and mix with a wooden spoon until combined. Stir in the chocolate chunks and bring the mixture together with your hands to form a dough.

Transfer the cookie dough to a large sheet of clingfilm, then roll into a wide 7cm (2¾ inch) sausage shape and wrap in the clingfilm, twisting the ends to seal. Chill in the refrigerator for 30 minutes.

Preheat the oven to 180°C/350°F/Gas Mark 4 and line 2 large baking sheets with baking paper.

Slice the dough into twelve 1.5cm- (⅝-inch-) thick discs and place, spaced well apart, on the prepared baking sheets. Bake for 10–12 minutes, or until golden brown around the edge and slightly paler in the centre.

Leave on the baking sheets for 2 minutes, then transfer to a wire rack to cool completely. The cookies will keep in an airtight container for up to 3 days.

Grilled pineapple with granita

Serves 6
1 pineapple, about 750g (1lb 10oz)
75g (2¾oz) palm sugar or dark brown soft sugar

For the granita:
250g (9oz) granulated sugar
500ml (18fl oz) cold water
4 strips of lime zest
4 large mint sprigs, bruised
250ml (9fl oz) lime juice (from about 6 large limes)
50ml (2fl oz) vodka

Begin by making the granita. Place the sugar, measured water and lime zest in a saucepan over a low heat. Heat gently to dissolve the sugar, then increase the heat to medium and bring to the boil. Simmer for 5 minutes, then remove from the heat and stir in the mint. Leave to cool, then strain.

Stir the lime juice and vodka into the sugar syrup and transfer to a freezer-proof bowl. Place in the freezer for about 4 hours until frozen.

Remove from the freezer for 15 minutes to soften, then transfer to a food processor and blend for 30 seconds until the mixture is soft and pale. Freeze again if necessary. Top and tail the pineapple and place it on one end on a chopping board. Using a sharp knife, cut downwards to remove the skin, working your way around the pineapple. Quarter and core the pineapple, then cut the flesh into wedges. Thread on to 6 metal skewers, then dip in the sugar. Preheat the grill to medium and grill the pineapple skewers for 2–3 minutes on each side until golden. Cool slightly and serve with the granita.

Hazelnut meringue stack

Serves 8

4 egg whites

250g (9oz) caster sugar

1 teaspoon white wine vinegar

100g (3½oz) blanched hazelnuts, toasted and roughly chopped*

200ml (7fl oz) double cream

275g (9¾oz) raspberries

cocoa powder, for dusting

Preheat the oven to 150°C/300°F/Gas Mark 2 and line 3 baking sheets with nonstick baking paper.

Whisk the egg whites in a large clean bowl until they form stiff peaks. Add the sugar, a spoonful at a time, and continue to whisk until thick and glossy. Fold in the vinegar with a large metal spoon.

Fold half the hazelnuts into the mixture, then divide it between the prepared sheets, spooning the meringue into 3 rounds roughly 18cm (7 inch) in diameter.

Bake for 45 minutes, then switch off the oven and leave the meringues inside to cool.

Whip the cream in a bowl until it forms soft peaks, then spoon it over 2 of the cooled meringues. Top each one with the raspberries and remaining nuts, reserving a few raspberries for decoration.

Stack the meringues with the plain one on top, then dust with a little cocoa powder and decorate with the remaining raspberries. Serve on the same day or chill for up to 2 days.

Lemon & poppy seed cupcakes

Makes 12

225g (8oz) gluten-free plain flour
2 teaspoons gluten-free baking powder
¼ teaspoon bicarbonate of soda
½ teaspoon salt
125g (4½oz) caster sugar
finely grated zest of 2 lemons and 1 tablespoon lemon juice
1 tablespoon poppy seeds, plus 1 teaspoon for decorating
75ml (2½fl oz) sunflower oil
7 tablespoons rice milk

For the frosting:

125g (4½oz) unsalted butter
250g (9oz) icing sugar
finely grated zest of 1 lemon
a few drops of yellow food colouring

Preheat the oven to 160°C/325°F/Gas Mark 3 and line a 12-hole cupcake tin with paper cases.

Sift the flour, baking powder, bicarbonate of soda and salt together in a large bowl. Stir in the sugar, lemon zest and poppy seeds.

In a jug, mix together the oil, rice milk and lemon juice. Add to the dry ingredients and stir to combine. Spoon the batter evenly into the prepared paper cases and bake for 15 minutes until just firm to the touch. Leave to cool on a wire rack.

To make the frosting, beat the butter, icing sugar, lemon zest and food colouring together in an electric mixer or in a bowl until soft and smooth. Spoon or pipe the frosting on to the cooled cakes and sprinkle with the remaining poppy seeds.

The cupcakes will keep in an air tight container for up to 3 days.

Lime & coconut cupcakes

Makes 12
125g (4½oz) softened unsalted butter
125g (4½oz) caster sugar
finely grated zest and juice of 2 limes
2 eggs
150g (5½oz) gluten-free self-raising flour
1 teaspoon gluten-free baking powder
50g (1¾oz) desiccated coconut*

For the frosting:
grated zest and juice of 1 lime
175g (6oz) icing sugar
a few drops of green food colouring
desiccated coconut, to decorate

Preheat the oven to 180°C/350°F/Gas Mark 4. Line a 12-hole cupcake tin with paper cases. In a large bowl, beat together the butter, caster sugar and lime zest with a hand-held electric whisk until pale and fluffy.

Beat in the eggs and lime juice, then fold in the flour, baking powder and desiccated coconut. Divide the mixture between the prepared paper cases. Bake for 15–20 minutes until risen and golden. Leave to cool on a wire rack.

To make the frosting, mix together the lime zest and juice with the icing sugar and food colouring in a bowl. Spoon over the cakes and sprinkle with the desiccated coconut.

The cupcakes will keep in an airtight container for up to 3 days.

Mandarin Eton mess

Makes 6 | Moderate-FODMAP recipe
360ml (12½fl oz) double cream
1 teaspoon finely grated orange zest (optional)
75g (2¾oz) ready-made meringues, broken into pieces
2 × 300g (10½oz) cans mandarin segments in juice, drained

In a large bowl, whip the cream with the orange zest, if using, until soft peaks form. Fold in the meringue pieces and mandarin segments, reserving a little of each to scatter over the top.

Spoon the mixture into bowls or sundae-style glasses and serve, scattered with the reserved meringue pieces and mandarin.

Rhubarb & raspberry crumble

Serves 4
500g (1lb 2oz) rhubarb, sliced
125g (4½oz) raspberries

50g (1¾oz) soft light brown sugar
3 tablespoons orange juice
lactose-free ice cream, to serve

For the crumble topping:
200g (7oz) gluten-free plain flour
pinch of salt
150g (5½oz) unsalted butter, diced
50g (1¾oz) soft light brown sugar

Preheat the oven to 200°C/400°F/Gas Mark 6 and grease a rectangular ovenproof dish.

Begin by making the crumble topping. Combine the flour and salt in a bowl, then add the butter and rub it in with your fingertips until the mixture resembles breadcrumbs. Stir in the sugar.

In a separate bowl, mix together the rhubarb, raspberries, sugar and orange juice, then tip into the prepared dish. Sprinkle over the topping and bake for about 25 minutes or until golden brown and bubbling.

Serve the crumble hot with a scoop of ice cream.

Sweet orange pancakes

Serves 4
200g (7oz) gluten-free plain flour
2 eggs
300ml (½ pint) lactose-free or plant-based milk (such as coconut, hemp, quinoa, rice, almond or hazelnut)
½ tablespoon sunflower oil, for oiling
2 oranges, zest grated and flesh segmented, juice reserved
2–3 tablespoons caster sugar, to serve

Sift the flour into a large bowl and make a well in the centre.

Add the eggs and whisk, using a hand-held electric whisk, then continue to whisk as you gradually add the milk and bring the flour from around the edges of the bowl into the batter. Once combined, leave to stand for 10 minutes.

Heat a small frying pan over a medium heat. Lightly oil the pan by wiping it with an oiled piece of kitchen paper.

Pour a generous tablespoon of the batter into the pan and tilt the pan to completely coat the base. Cook the pancake for 3–4 minutes, then turn over and cook the other side for 2–3 minutes.

Transfer the pancake to a plate lined with baking paper and keep warm. Repeat with the remaining batter to make 8 pancakes.

Pour the orange juice into a separate pan over a low heat. Add the orange segments and zest and warm through. Pour this mixture over the pancakes and sprinkle with sugar, then serve.

Vanilla & jam shortbread

Makes 8

125g (4½oz) unsalted butter

50g (1¾oz) caster sugar

150g (5½oz) gluten-free plain flour, plus extra for dusting

25g (1oz) cornflour

1 teaspoon vanilla extract

3 tablespoons raspberry or strawberry jam (choose a variety that is made with 100 per cent fruit)

icing sugar, for dusting

In an electric mixer, beat together the butter and sugar until pale and fluffy. Sift the flour and cornflour into the mixture, then add the vanilla. Mix until combined. Roll the dough into a ball, then wrap in clingfilm and chill for 30 minutes.

Preheat the oven to 160°C/325°F/Gas Mark 3 and line 2 baking sheets with baking paper.

On a lightly floured surface, roll out the dough to a thickness of about 5mm (¼ inch). Use a 5cm (2 inch) square or round cutter to cut out 16 squares or rounds, rerolling the trimmings as necessary. Place the cut out pieces on the prepared baking sheets and bake for 10–12 minutes until pale golden.

Leave the shortbreads to cool on the baking sheets for 10 minutes until firm, then transfer to a wire rack to cool completely. Sandwich the biscuits together with the jam and dust with icing sugar.

The shortbread will keep in an airtight container for up to 3 days.

CONCLUSION

The low-FODMAP diet is a wonderful tool that can have amazing results for many people (although, as I have explained, it is not a magic cure and sadly will not work for everyone). To succeed with this diet, you really do need access to a dietitian and support from those around you. It takes time, preparation, food knowledge and sticking power. If the low-FODMAP diet is not for you, there are modified approaches and other options, so do not give up: ask, ask, and ask again for more help and support. It could be your IBS has been misdiagnosed or that you need another strategy.

IBS is a complex and misunderstood condition, often with a stigma attached to it. It is very real and not something to be ignored or pushed aside. Taking the time to understand your body and get connected to your digestive system can be so very worthwhile. I hope that by going on this journey, you don't just learn more about your IBS, but about yourself too.

Please remember that this book is not the IBS Bible: it's here to provide education and act as a resource while you work with your medical team.

RESOURCES

Apps

There are a number of good apps that you can use to help manage your stress levels, track your IBS symptoms, monitor your reintroductions or check a food's FODMAP content.

Nerva provides a six-week psychology-based programme taking you through gut-directed hypnotherapy. This can provide you with techniques to reduce the pain signals and symptoms.

Bowelle enables you to track your food intake and symptoms, which can help you see which foods are causing issues. It's also useful to show to your dietitian. The app allows you to add your menstrual cycle and monitor stressful events, which will also help you see patterns and links.

The Monash University FODMAP Diet app is an essential app to help you identify how much of certain foods you can eat. It uses a traffic-light system showing foods as red (high in FODMAPs), amber (medium) or green (low). You can use the food diary to record your diet and symptoms, plus any stress you may be experiencing. There are recipes and a reintroductions diary to use to record your symptoms as you challenge different foods.

FODMAP by FM is a UK-based app that has a barcode scanner you can use to check foods for their FODMAP content. You can track your reintroductions and share this information with your dietitian, using use it to create your own personalized modified FODMAP diet.

Calm is a popular meditation app that includes guided meditations and tips on mindful movement.

Headspace is a meditation and mindfulness app designed to help you reduce and manage stress levels.

Insight Timer is a meditation app with a variety of guided mediations.

Websites
IBS Network
The UK's national charity offering information, advice and support to patients with IBS. Members of the network also have access to their team of IBS specialists, including gastroenterologists, specialist dietitians and pharmacists through their Ask the Experts service, and to IBS-trained nurses through their helpline.
www.theibsnetwork.org / 0114 272 3253

Guts UK

A UK charity funding research into and raising awareness of various digestive issues.

www.gutscharity.org.uk

Clinical Alimentary

Dietary advice and resources for people with IBS.

www.clinicalalimentary.blog

King's College London

The home of King's College London's extensive research into FODMAPs and digestive health.

www.kcl.ac.uk/lsm/Schools/life-course-sciences/departments/nutritional-sciences/projects/fodmaps

Monash University

Detailed information about IBS and FODMAPs from one of the area's leading research groups.

www.monashfodmap.com

Shepherd Works

Nutritional advice and support for people with IBS, gluten intolerance and coeliac disease.

www.shepherdworks.com.au

A Little Bit Yummy

Low-FODMAP recipes and resources.

www.alittlebityummy.com

Fodmap Everyday

Recipes and resources for people on a low-FODMAP diet.

www.fodmapeveryday.com

My GI Nutrition

Advice and information about symptoms, FODMAPs and the low-FODMAP diet.

www.myginutrition.com

Kate Scarlata

Kate is a Boston-based dietitian who has a wealth of FODMAP resources on her website.

www.katescarlata.com

Somerset Partnership NHS Trust Low-FODMAP Webinar

A one-hour long webinar full of detailed information from a specialist team of NHS dietitians.

www.youtube.com/watch?v=m1U7NyBBbT0

Books

IBS and FODMAPs

King's College London FODMAP booklets (ask your dietitian for copies)

The Low FODMAP Recipe Book by Lucy Whigam (Aster, 2017)

The Complete Low FODMAP Diet by Dr Sue Shepherd and Dr Peter Gibson (Vermillion, 2014)

The Low FODMAP Diet Cookbook by Dr Sue Shepherd (Vermillion, 2015)

The Low FODMAP Diet by Penny Doyle (Lorenz Books, 2015)

Eat Yourself Healthy by Dr Megan Rossi (Penguin Life, 2019)

Mindfulness, meditation and lifestyle

Mindfulness by Professor Mark Williams and Dr Danny Penman (Piatkus Books, 2011)

The 4 Pillar Plan by Dr Ranjan Chatterjee (Penguin Life, 2018)

Ready meals

Field Doctor

A range of low-FODMAP ready meals designed by a dietitian.

www.fielddoctor.co.uk

Bay's Kitchen

Low-FODMAP sauces, soups and stocks.

www.bayskitchen.com

Where to find a dietitian

Worldwide

The Monash University website has a list of dietitians who have completed the Monash FODMAP course. This is the main course that dietitians complete to be FODMAP-trained and you can find dietitians here from around the world:

www.monashfodmap.com/online-training/fodmap-dietitians-directory/

Fodmap Everyday List

A global directory of registered dietitians who have experience with the low-FODMAP diet.

www.fodmapeveryday.com/resources/registered-dietitian-directory/

UK

Freelance Dietitians

A directory of UK-based freelance dietitians with a range of specialities.

https://freelancedietitians.org

US

Eat Right: Academy of Nutrition and Dietetics

A directory of registered dietitians in the US.

www.eatright.org/find-a-nutrition-expert

REFERENCES

1 Shepherd S.J., Gibson P.R., 2006, 'Fructose malabsorption and symptoms of irritable bowel syndrome: guidelines for effective dietary management.' *Journal of the American Dietetic Association*, 106 (10), pp. 1631–9. doi: 10.1016/j.jada.2006.07.010. PMID: 17000196.

2 Gibson P.R., Shepherd S.J., 2010, 'Evidence-based dietary management of functional gastrointestinal symptoms: The FODMAP approach.' *Journal of Gastroenterology and Hepatology*, 25 (2), pp. 252–8.

3 McKenzie Y.A., et al, 2016. 'British Dietetic Association systematic review and evidence-based practice guidelines for the dietary management of irritable bowel syndrome in adults' (2016 update). *Journal of Human Nutrition and Dietetics*, 29, pp. 549–575.

4 Whelan K., Martin L.D., Staudacher H.M., Lomer M.C.E., 2018, 'The low-FODMAP diet in the management of irritable bowel syndrome: An evidence-based review of FODMAP restriction, reintroduction and personalisation in clinical practice.' *Journal of Human Nutrition and Dietetics*, 31 (2), pp. 239–255. doi: 10.1111/jhn.12530.

5 National Institute for Health and Care Excellence [NICE], 2008. *Irritable bowel syndrome in adults: diagnosis and management.* (NICE Guideline No. CG61). www.nice.org.u/guidajce/cg61.

6 Lovell R.M., Ford A.C., 2012, 'Global prevalence of and risk factors for irritable bowel syndrome: a meta-analysis.' *Clinical Gastroenterology and Hepatology*, 10 (7), pp. 712–721.

7 Hungin, A.P., et al., 2003, 'The prevalence, patterns and impact of irritable bowel syndrome: an international survey of 40,000 subjects.' *Alimentary Pharmacology and Therapeutics*, 17 (5), pp. 643–50.

8 NICE, 2008, *Irritable bowel syndrome in adults.*

9 ROME IV Criteria: https://theromefoundation.org/rome-iv/rome-iv-criteria/

10 NICE, 2008, *Irritable bowel syndrome in adults.*

11 Marshall J.K., Thabane M., Garg A.X., et al., 2010, 'Eight-year prognosis of postinfectious irritable bowel syndrome following waterborne bacterial dysentery.' *Gut*, 59 (5), pp. 605–611. doi: 10.1136/gut.2009.202234.

12 Gibson P.R., Shepherd S.J. 2010. 'Evidence-based dietary management of functional gastrointestinal symptoms.'

13 McKenzie Y.A., et al (2016). 'British Dietetic Association systematic review and evidence-based practise guidelines.'

14 McKenzie Y.A., et al (2016). 'British Dietetic Association systematic review and evidence-based practise guidelines.'

15 McKenzie Y.A., et al (2016). 'British Dietetic Association systematic review and evidence-based practise guidelines.'

16 McKenzie Y.A., et al (2016). 'British Dietetic Association systematic review and evidence-based practise guidelines'.

17 McKenzie Y.A., et al (2016). 'British Dietetic Association systematic review and evidence-based practise guidelines'.

18 McKenzie Y.A., et al (2016). 'British Dietetic Association systematic review and evidence-based practise guidelines'.

19 McKenzie Y.A., et al (2016). 'British Dietetic Association systematic review and evidence-based practise guidelines'.

20 NICE, 2008, *Irritable bowel syndrome in adults*.

21 NICE, 2008, *Irritable bowel syndrome in adults*.

22 Gill S.K., Rossi M., Bajka B., Whelan K., 2021, 'Dietary fibre in gastrointestinal health and disease.' *Nature Reviews Gastroenterology and Hepatology*, 18 (2), pp. 101–116. doi: 10.1038/s41575-020-00375-4. PMID: 33208922.

23 Agrawal A., Houghton L.A., Morris J., Reilly B., Guyonnet D., Goupil Feuillerat N., Schlumberger A., Jakob S., Whorwell P.J., 2009, 'Clinical trial: the effects of a fermented milk product containing *Bifidobacterium lactis* DN-173 010 on abdominal distension and gastrointestinal transit in irritable bowel syndrome with constipation.' *Alimentary Pharmacology and Therapeutics*, 29 (1), pp.104–14. doi: 10.1111/j.1365-2036.2008.03853.x. PMID: 18801055.

24 Sisson G., Ayis S., Sherwood R.A., Bjarnason I., 2014, 'Randomised clinical trial: A liquid multi-strain probiotic vs. placebo in the irritable bowel syndrome – a 12 week double-blind study.' *Alimentary Pharmacology and Therapeutics*, 40 (1), pp. 51–62. doi: 10.1111/apt.12787. Epub 2014 May 11. PMID: 24815298.

25 O'Mahony L., McCarthy J., Kelly P., Hurley G., Luo F., Chen K., O'Sullivan G. C., Kiely B., Collins J. K., Shanahan F., Quigley E.M., 2005, 'Lactobacillus and bifidobacterium in irritable bowel syndrome: symptom responses and relationship to cytokine profiles.' *Gastroenterology*, 128 (3), pp. 541–51. doi: 10.1053/j. gastro.2004.11.050. PMID: 15765388.

26 Kim H. J., Vazquez Roque M. I., Camilleri M., Stephens D., Burton D. D., Baxter K., Thomforde G., Zinsmeister A. R., 2005, 'A randomized controlled trial of a probiotic combination VSL# 3 and placebo in irritable bowel syndrome with bloating.' *Neurogastroenterolgy and Motility*, 17 (5), pp. 687–96. doi: 10.1111/j.1365-2982.2005.00695.x. PMID: 16185307.

27 NICE, 2008, *Irritable bowel syndrome in adults*.

28 Schumann D., Anheyer D., Lauche R., Dobos G., Langhorst J., Cramer H., 2016, 'Effect of Yoga in the Therapy of Irritable Bowel Syndrome: A Systematic Review.' *Clinical Gastroenterology and Hepatology*, 14 (12), pp. 1720–1731. doi: 10.1016/j. cgh.2016.04.026. PMID: 27112106.

29 Böhn L. et al., 2012, 'Nutrient intake in patients with irritable bowel syndrome compared with the general population.' *Neurogastroenterology and Motility*, 25 (1), p.23.

30 Böhn L., Storsrud S., Liljebo T., et al., 2015, 'A diet low in FODMAPs reduces symptoms of irritable bowel syndrome as well as traditional dietary advice: A randomized controlled trial.' *Gastroenterology*, 149 (6), pp. 1399–1407.

31   Dionne J., Ford A., Yuan Y., et al., 2018, 'A systematic review and meta-analysis evaluating the efficacy of a gluten-free diet and a low-FODMAPs diet in treating symptoms of irritable bowel syndrome.' *American Journal of Gastroenterology*, 113 (9), pp.1290–1300.

32   Eswaran S.L., Chey W.D., Han-Markey T., Ball S., Jackson K., 2016, 'A randomized controlled trial comparing the low-FOD-MAP diet vs. modified NICE guidelines in US adults with IBS-D.' *American Journal of Gastroenterology*, 111 (12), pp.1824–1832. doi: 10.1038/ajg.2016.434.

33   Shepherd S.J., Gibson P.R., 2006, 'Fructose malabsorption'.

34   Eswaran S.L. et al., 2016, 'A randomized controlled trial comparing the low-FODMAP diet vs. modified NICE guidelines in US adults with IBS-D.'

35   Staudacher H.M., Whelan K., 2017, 'The low-FODMAP diet: Recent advances in understanding its mechanisms and efficacy in IBS.' *Gut*, 66 (8) p. 1517. doi: 10.1136/gutjnl-2017-313750.

36   Staudacher H.M., Whelan K., 2017, 'The low-FODMAP diet: Recent advances in understanding'.

37   Major G., Pritchard S., Murray K., et al., 2017, 'Colon hypersensitivity to distension, rather than excessive gas production, produces carbohydrate-related symptoms in individuals with irritable bowel syndrome.' *Gastroenterology*, 152 (1), pp.124–133.

38   Ong D.K., Mitchell S.B., Barrett J.S., et al., 2010, 'Manipulation of dietary short-chain carbohydrates alters the pattern of gas production and genesis of symptoms in irritable bowel syndrome.' *Journal of Gastroenterology and Hepatology*, 25 (8), p.1366.

39 Staudacher H.M., Whelan K., 2017, 'The low-FODMAP diet: Recent advances in understanding'.

40 Staudacher H.M., Whelan K., 2017, 'The low-FODMAP diet: Recent advances in understanding'.

41 McKenzie Y.A., et al (2016). 'British Dietetic Association systematic review and evidence-based practise guidelines'.

42 Halmos E.P., Power V.A., Shepherd S.J., et al., 2014, 'A diet low in FODMAPs reduces symptoms of irritable bowel syndrome.' *Gastroenterology*, 146 (1), pp.67–75.

43 Staudacher H.M., Lomer M.C.E., Louis P., et al., 2016, 'The low-FODMAP diet reduces symptoms in irritable bowel syndrome compared with placebo diet and the microbiota alterations may be prevented by probiotic co-administration: A 2x2 factorial randomised controlled trial.' *Gastroenterology*, 150 (4), p.S230.

44 Farrokhyar F., Marshall J.K., Easterbrook B., Irvine E.J., 2006, 'Functional gastrointestinal disorders and mood disorders in patients with inactive inflammatory bowel disease: prevalence and impact on health.' *Inflammatory Bowel Diseases*, 12 (1), pp.38–46.

45 Farrokhyar F., Marshall J.K., Easterbrook B., Irvine E.J., 2006, 'Functional gastrointestinal disorders and mood disorders'.

46 Gearry R.B., Irving P.M., Barrett J.S., Nathan D.M., Shepherd S.J., Gibson P.R., 2009, 'Reduction of dietary poorly absorbed short-chain carbohydrates (FODMAPs) improves abdominal symptoms in patients with inflammatory bowel disease: A pilot study.' *Journal of Crohn's and Colitis*, 3 (1), pp. 8–14.

47 Gibson P.R., Shepherd S.J., 2010, 'Evidence-based dietary management of functional gastrointestinal symptoms'.

48 Barrett J.S., Gearry R.B., Muir J.G., Irving P.M., Rose R., Rosella O., Haines M.L., Shepherd S.J., Gibson P.R., 2010, 'Dietary poorly absorbed, short-chain carbohydrates increase delivery of water and fermentable substrates to the proximal colon.' *Alimentary Pharmacology and Therapeutics*, 31 (8), pp. 874–82.

49 McKenzie Y.A., et al (2016). 'British Dietetic Association systematic review and evidence-based practise guidelines'.

50 Whelan K., et al (2018). 'The low-FODMAP diet in the management of irritable bowel syndrome'.

51 Shepherd S.J, Gibson P.R., 2006, 'Fructose malabsorption'.

52 McKenzie Y.A., et al (2016). 'British Dietetic Association systematic review and evidence-based practise guidelines'.

53 Whelan K., et al (2018). 'The low-FODMAP diet in the management of irritable bowel syndrome'.

54 McKenzie Y.A., et al (2016). 'British Dietetic Association systematic review and evidence-based practise guidelines'.

55 Whelan K., et al (2018). 'The low-FODMAP diet in the management of irritable bowel syndrome'.

56 Halmos E.P., Christophersen C.T., Bird A.R., Shepherd S.J., Muir J.G., Gibson P.R., 2016, 'Consistent Prebiotic Effect on Gut Microbiota With Altered FODMAP Intake in Patients with Crohn's Disease: A Randomised, Controlled Cross-Over Trial of Well-Defined Diets.' *Clinical and Translational Gastroenterology*, 7 (4), p. 164. doi: 10.1038/ctg.2016.22. PMID: 27077959; PMCID: PMC4855163.

57 Staudacher H.M., Lomer M.C., Anderson J.L., et al., 2012, 'Fermentable carbohydrate restriction reduces luminal *bifidobacteria* and gastrointestinal symptoms in patients with irritable bowel syndrome.' *Journal of Nutrition*, 142 (8), pp. 1510–8.

58 McKenzie Y.A., et al (2016). 'British Dietetic Association systematic review and evidence-based practise guidelines'.

59 Staudacher H.M., Lomer M.C.E., Farquharson F.M., et al., 2017, 'A diet low in FODMAPs reduces symptoms in patients with irritable bowel syndrome and a probiotic restores *Bifidobacterium* species: A randomized controlled trial.' *Gastroenterology*, 153 (4), pp. 936–947.

60 Staudacher H.M., et al., 2017, 'A diet low in FODMAPs reduces symptoms in patients with irritable bowel syndrome'.

61 Staudacher H.M., et al., 2012, 'Fermentable carbohydrate restriction'.

62 Wilson B., Rossi M., Dimidi E., Whelan K., 2019, 'Prebiotics in irritable bowel syndrome and other functional bowel disorders in adults: A systematic review and meta-analysis of randomized controlled trials.' *American Journal of Clinical Nutrition*, 109 (4), pp. 1098–1111. doi: 10.1093/ajcn/nqy376.

63 Wilson B., Rossi M., Kanno T., et al., 2020, 'β-Galactooligosaccharide in Conjunction With Low-FODMAP Diet Improves Irritable Bowel Syndrome Symptoms but Reduces Fecal Bifidobacteria.' *American Journal of Gastroenterology*, 115 (6), pp. 906–915. doi:10.14309/ajg.0000000000000641.

UK terms and their US equivalents

aubergine	eggplant	haricot beans	navy beans
baking paper	parchment paper or wax paper	icing sugar	confectioners' sugar/ powdered sugar
baking tin	baking pan	kitchen paper	paper towels
beef fillet	beef tenderloin	lamb mince	ground lamb
beef mince	ground beef	mangetout	snow peas
beetroot	beets	muffin tin	muffin pan
biscuits	cookies	natural yogurt	plain yogurt
broad beans	fava beans	pak choi	bok choy
butter beans	lima beans	peppers (red/ green/yellow)	bell peppers
cake tin	cake pan	plain flour	all-purpose flour
cannellini beans	white kidney beans	pork mince	ground pork
caster sugar	superfine sugar	porridge oats	rolled oats/ oatmeal
celeriac	celery root	roasting tray	roasting pan
chickpeas	garbanzo beans	self-raising flour	self-rising flour
Chinese leaf	nappa cabbage/ Chinese cabbage	sieve	fine mesh strainer
coriander (fresh)	cilantro	soured cream	sour cream
cornflour	cornstarch	spring onions	scallions
courgettes	zucchini	stock	broth
double cream	heavy cream	sultanas	golden raisins
golden syrup	*can substitute corn syrup*	swede	rutabaga
griddle pan	grill pan	long-stem broccoli	broccolini
grill	broiler	tomato purée	tomato paste

INDEX

THANKS

I'm a hugely spiritual person, so the biggest thanks goes to God, who literally sustains me. You are my rock.

To my parents, who have taught me that I can do anything I set my mind to. Thank you for always believing in me and for teaching me how to aim for the stars.

Huge love and thanks to Lucy and Rich, who have looked after my children when I needed to write, listened to my moaning and encouraged me to keep going.

Corrie, my agent: thank you for your support, for helping me to keep perspective and for telling me I could do this when I felt as though I couldn't.

Special thanks to some wonderful dietitians who have given me advice, read over parts of this book and been a sounding board.

Finally, thanks to the team at Octopus for making this book happen and for bringing it to life. Your expertise is invaluable and I'm so excited to see this book in the flesh!